SIRTFOOD DIET
FOR WOMEN

HEAL YOUR BODY WITH FOODS THAT TURN ON YOUR
SO-CALLED SKINNY GENES, CURE YOUR MIND WITH ENERGY
MEDICINE THERAPY TO INCREASE HAPPINESS,
CLARITY AND EMOTIONAL RESILIENCE.

Adele Young

Table of Contents

SIRTFOOD DIET

ADELE YOUNG

ADELE YOUNG

Introduction

Fasting-based diets have become very popular over the past few years. In fact, studies show that by fasting – that is, with moderate daily calorie restriction or by practising a more radical, but less frequent, intermittent fast – you can expect to lose about 3kg in six months and substantially reduce the risk of contracting certain diseases.

When we fast, the reduction of energy reserves activates the so-called "skinny gene", which causes several positive changes. The accumulation of fat stops and the body blocks normal growth processes and enters the "survival" mode. Fats burn faster, and the genes that repair and rejuvenate cells are activated. As a result, we lose weight and increase our resistance to diseases.

All this, however, has a price. Lower energy intake leads to hunger, irritability, exhaustion and loss of muscle mass and this is a problem, the main problem, with fasting-based diets: when they are followed correctly, they work, but they make us feel so bad that we cannot repeat them. The question, then, is the following: is it possible to obtain the same results without having to impose that drastic drop in calories and, therefore, without suffering the negative consequences?

According to the sirtfood diet, it is. In fact, there is a skinny gene that, if activated properly, allows you to lose weight and gain health altogether. The singer Adele has lost 30kg in a year thanks to this philosophy: a prog of two medical nutritionists, Aidan Goggins and Glen Matten, which is based on the introduction of some sirtfoods in our diet.

These are particularly nutrient-rich foods capable of activating the same skinny genes stimulated by fasting. These genes are called sirtuins and considered to be super regulators of metabolism to influence our ability to burn fat.

This book is your sirt diet know-it-all guide. It will guide you through fun and straightforward sirt recipes that will have you shedding fat daily.

Chapter 1:
What is a sirtfood?

The sirtfood diet focuses on ingredients experts say can help you live longer and turbocharge weight loss. These foods are full of components that activate the skinny gene sirtuins, which in turn revs up your weight loss. Sirtuins are a type of protein involved in regulating essential processes such as metabolism and cellular death. The breakthrough for this diet emerged when researchers discovered the benefits of fasting that come from the activation of our sirtuins gene.

When there is a shortage of energy, your body goes under stress detected by the sirtuins. The sirtuins then activate and subsequently broadcast strong signals that change the behaviour of our cells in a way that fosters a healthier, fitter, and leaner you.

"Sirtfood" is food with a high content of sirtuin activators. The word "sirt" in "sirtfood" is an abbreviation for the enzyme group of sirtuins.

While the popular low carb diet is full of proteins and allows only a small amount of carbohydrates, the sirt diet focuses on sirtuins. These are enzymes in the body that protect the cells in the body from stress through their unique activity, namely reducing the production of free radicals. If the body absorbs enough sirtuin activators from food, it also burns fat.

The advantage: sirtuin activators are contained in a wide variety of foods and beverages, including luxury foods, and thus enable a varied diet that is not very restrictive. The only task in this diet is to consume as many foods as possible that are rich in these sirtuin activators.

Sirtuins strengthen the immune system, help build muscle and ensure that cell metabolism decreases – in other words, the ageing process slows down, you stay "young longer". All you need to do is switch to foods that activate many sirtuins.

Sirtuins not only make you young and healthy but also slim. The promise of the sirtuin diet: within one week, you can lose up to 3kg. If you also exercise more and burn calories, you can become even slimmer in this short period; because the more muscles you have, the more calories you burn. Sirtuin-activating foods also inhibit ravenous appetite attacks.

The best-known woman that the sirt diet has helped is none other than singer Adele.

The sirtfood diet depends on the possibility that specific nourishments initiate sirtuins in your body, which are specific proteins conjectured to receive different rewards, from shielding cells in your body from aggravation to turning around maturing. Nourishments permitted on a diet incorporate green tea, dull chocolate, apples, natural citrus products, parsley, turmeric, kale, blueberries, tricks and red wine.

On the authority sirtfood diet site, defenders clarify that the diet has two "simple" stages. Stage one is seven days with every day comprising of three sirtfood green juices and one dinner loaded up with sirtfoods – an aggregate of 1,000 calories. Yet, don't be disheartened: you may be somewhat less starving on days four through seven when you're permitted to build your admission to 1,500 calories with two green juices and two dinners. Phew!

Stage two isn't considerably more encouraging. This stage goes on for about fourteen days, in which you are allowed to have three "adjusted" sirtfood-rich dinners every day notwithstanding your one unique green juice. The objective during this time is to advance further weight loss. While the advantages of sirtuins appear to be encouraging, the sirtfood diet is showcased up until now another approach to "shed seven pounds in seven days!" and you know at this point extreme diets simply don't work that way.

Here are three motivations to take a pass on the sirtfood diet:

1. The sirtfood diet estimates achievement just as far as weight loss.

Weight is a determinant of wellbeing, yet it's not alone. To gauge somebody's wellbeing accomplishment on whether they lose 'x' pounds in 'x' measure of time overlooks the various advantages of nourishment. Nourishment is brimming with vitality, which enables you to do things like showering, practising and relaxing. It additionally has supplements that can advance a few substantial capacities and is often a cheerful encounter established in custom. For by and large wellbeing, there's a great deal more to concentrate on than basically appearance, and estimating achievement just as far as weight loss is incomprehensive.

2. It's prohibitive, which can harm your association with nourishment.

This diet stresses an admission of 1,000 to 1,500 calories for every day, which is a lot of lower than a great many people need. When we seriously limit our nourishment admission, our intuitive response is to indulge. Your body is savvy, and it thinks about this absence of sustenance as an assault. Therefore, we will in general overcompensate, which is the reason we as a whole can identify with being "hangry" and thus overindulging when we're at last allowed to eat. Rehearsing careful and intuitive eating is a more practical course than confining nourishment.

3. The sirtfood diet isn't science-based.

While there is some questionable research about the advantages of sirtuins, there's practically zero research about the specific sirtfood diet. Moreover, we, as of now, have a few rules set up that have been thoroughly looked into and tried for quite a long time. If you're lost on what "sound nourishment" is, this is a superior spot to begin.

It's fine if you need to join a couple sirtfoods into an eating plan. Nourishments like green tea, organic product, dim chocolate and kale all include a spot inside a smart dieting design! Be that as it may, holding fast to a prog with such exacting pass-or-bomb prerequisites is unreasonable and could be hurtful to your association with nourishment. By fusing an eating plan that is loaded with assortment and eating carefully, you'll have the option to set up a long haul, manageable association with nourishment. Cheers to that!

What to know before start sirtfood diet

"Sirtfood" seems like something created by outsiders, brought to earth for human utilisation with expectations of picking up mind control and global control. In fact, sirtfoods are essentially nourishments high in sirtuins. Uh, come again? Sirtuins are a sort of protein that reviews on natural product flies, and mice have indicated control digestion, increment bulk and consume fat.

As indicated by the book, this arrangement can assist you with consuming fat and lift your vitality, preparing your body for long haul weight-loss achievement and a more drawn out more beneficial ailment free life and all that while drinking red wine. Sounds like practically the ideal diet, isn't that so? All things considered, before you consume your reserve funds loading up on sirtuins-filled fixings, read the upsides and downsides.

The underlying power of sirtfoods

Sirtfoods are simply foods that activate the sirtuin genes. These foods are unique for this function because they contain a natural plant chemical known as polyphenols. This chemical 'speaks' to the sirtuin genes and switches them on. Polyphenols are dietary antioxidants that help decrease the development of fat cells and reduce fatty tissue – they mimic the effects of fasting or exercising.

Because they are stationary, plants have developed a sophisticated stress response system. They produce polyphenols to help them adapt to harsh environments. By consuming these plants, we benefit from the effects that activate our innate stress response pathways.

All plants have these response systems, but only certain plants produce a significant amount of the sirtuin-activating polyphenol. Discovery of these foods means you can lose weight through eating sirtfoods.

What is so great about sirtuins?

There are seven types of sirtuins named from *sirt1* to *sirt7*. Although our understanding of the exact functions of all the sirtuins is minimal, studies show that activating them can have the following benefits:

- *Switching on fat burning and protection from weight gain:* sirtuins do this by increasing the functionality of the mitochondrion (which is involved in the production of energy) and sparking a change in your metabolism to break down more fat cells.

- The activated sirts increase the amount of a neurotransmitter known as norepinephrine used as a signal to fat cells. These transmitters tell the fat cells to breakdown fat and convert into energy.

- *Improving memory* by protecting neurons from damage. Sirtuins also boost learning skills and memory through the enhancement of synaptic plasticity. Synaptic plasticity refers to the ability of synapses to weaken or strengthen with time due to decrease or increase in their activity. This is important because memories are represented by different interconnect network of synapses in the brain and synaptic plasticity is an important neurochemical foundation of memory and learning.

- *Slowing down the ageing process:* sirtuins act as cell guarding enzymes. Thus, they protect the cells and slow down their ageing process.

- *Repairing cells:* the sirtuins repair cells damaged by re-activating cell functionality.

- *Protection against diabetes:* this happens through prevention against insulin resistance. Sirtuins do this by controlling blood sugar levels because this diet calls for moderate consumption of carbohydrates. These foods cause increases in blood sugar levels; hence the need to release insulin and as the blood sugar levels increase greatly there is need to produce more insulin. Over time, cells become resistant to insulin; hence, the need to produce more insulin and this leads to insulin resistance.

- *Fighting cancers:* the chemicals working as sirtuin activators affect the function of sirtuin in different cells, *i.e.* By switching it on when in normal cells and shutting it down in cancerous cells. This encourages the death of cancerous cells.

- *Fighting inflammation:* sirtuins have a powerful antioxidant effect that has the power to reduce oxidative stress. This has positive effects on heart health and cardiovascular protection.

Food list

Sirtfoods list in addition to red wine and chocolate allowed in this diet, here are other foods included:

Apples	Coffee	Onions	Strawberries
Blueberries	Dates	Parsley	Tofu
Capers	Fruits and	Passion fruit	Turmeric
Celery	Kale	Red chicory	Vegetables
Chilli	Lovage	Rocket	Walnuts
Citrus fruits	Medjool	Soy	

Red wine in this diet steals the limelight because it is rich in sirtuins and because it is most people's favourite type of drink.

chocolate contains sirtuin-activating antioxidant resveratrol. You should opt for dark chocolate rather than milk chocolate, however, for the greatest benefit, opt for baking chocolate or cocoa powder, which contain more resveratrol than all ready to eat chocolates.

Olive oil has a sufficient amount of the sirt activator oleuropein. To get the best out of olive oil, use extra virgin olive oil (EVOO). The benefits of the oil start at 2 tbsp a day.

Green tea contains a phytochemical known as epigallocatechin-3-gallate (egcg) known to activate and control sirtuins directly to anti-cancer action. Preferably, drink matcha green ta because it contains three times more egcg than other brands of green tea.

Now that you know what the sirtfood diet is, the function of sirtuins, how sirtuins help the body lose weight, as well as the foods you should reach for, the rest of the guide shall revolve around giving you easy and delicious sirtfood diet recipes.

The taste does not tell us which food contains sirtuin – it is found in bitter fruits and vegetables as well as in sweets. For this reason, we have created a small overview of foods that contain sirtuin.

Of course, you do not have to limit yourself to the following list of foods. The aim is to include the delicacies containing sirtuin in the menu as often as possible. For luxury goods such as coffee, chocolate or red wine, the following applies: always enjoy with care and do not eat or drink too much.

20 most important sirtfoods:

Arugula	Cocoa (pure or in 85% chocolate)	Lovage	Soya
Buckwheat		Olive oil	Strawberries
Capers	Coffee	Onions (red)	Turmeric
Celery	Dates (Medjoul)	Parsley	Walnuts
Chillies (birds eye chilli)	Green tea	Radicchio	
	Kale	Red wine	

The following 40 other sirtuin-activating foods are also recommended in the sirtfood diet. These are not quite as strongly activating as those from the top 20 list but are still highly recommended.

Fruits

• apples • blackberries • cranberries • goji berries • raspberries • currants (black) • kumquats • plums • grapes (red)

Vegetables and legumes

• artichokes • broccoli • watercress • chicory (light) • broad beans • white beans • green beans • last salad • bok choy • shallots • asparagus • onions (white)

Beverages

• black tea • white tea

Cereals

• popcorn • quinoa • wholemeal flour

Herbs and spices

• chilli • dill • ginger • mint • oregano • legend • chives • thyme

Nuts and seeds

chia seeds • peanuts • chestnuts • pecan nuts • pistachios • sunflower seeds

How can it work?

At its centre, the way to getting in shape is really basic: create a calorie shortage either by expanding your calorie consume exercises or diminishing your caloric admission. Be that as it may, imagine a scenario where you could avoid the dieting and rather actuate a "thin quality" without the requirement for extraordinary calorie limitation. This is the reason for the sirtfood diet, composed by nourishment specialists Aidan Goggins and Glen Matten. The best approach to do it, they contend, is sirtfoods.

Sirtfoods are wealthy in supplements that enact a purported "thin quality" called sirtuin. As indicated by Goggins and Matten, the "thin quality" is enacted when a lack of vitality is made after you confine calories. Sirtuins got intriguing to the sustenance world in 2003 when scientists found that resveratrol, a compound found in red wine, had a similar impact on life length as calorie limitation yet it was accomplished without decreasing admission. (Discover the conclusive truth about wine and its medical advantages.)

In the 2015 pilot study (led by Goggins and Matten) testing the adequacy of sirtuins, the 39 members lost a normal of seven pounds in seven days. Those outcomes sound amazing, yet it's imperative to understand this is a small example size concentrated over a brief timeframe. Weight-loss specialists additionally have their questions about the elevated guarantees. "The cases made are theoretical and extrapolate from considers which were generally centred around straightforward creatures (like yeast) at the cell level. What occurs at the cell level doesn't mean what occurs in the human body at the large scale level," says Adrienne Youdim, m.d., the chief of the Centre for Weight Loss and Nutrition in Beverly Hills, CA. (Here, look at the best and most exceedingly awful diets to follow this year.)

The diet is executed in two stages. Stage one endures three days and limits calories to 1,000 every day, comprising of three green juices and one sirtfood-endorsed supper. Stage two keeps going four days and raises the everyday designation to 1,500 calories for each day with two green juices and two dinners.

After these stages, there is an upkeep plan that isn't centred around calories yet rather on reasonable bits, well-adjusted suppers, and topping off on principally sirtfoods. The 14-day upkeep plan highlights three dinners, one green juice, and a couple sirtfood chomp snacks. Adherents are additionally urged to finish 30 minutes of movement five days per week-per government proposals; however, it isn't the fundamental focal point of the arrangement.

What are the advantages?

You will get thinner if you follow this diet intently. "Regardless of whether you're eating 1,000 calories of tacos, 1,000 calories of kale, or 1,000 calories of snickerdoodles, you will get in shape at 1,000 calories!" says dr. Youdim. In any case, she additionally calls attention to that you can have accomplishment with an increasingly sensible calorie limitation. "The run of the mill every day caloric admission of somebody not on a diet is 2,000 to 2,200, so lessening to 1,500 is as yet limiting and would be a powerful weight-loss procedure for most," she says.

Sirtfood Allergy labels:

Sf – soy-free   Ef – egg-free

Gf – gluten-free   V – vegan

Df – dairy-free   Nf – nut-free

Are there any safeguards?

"This arrangement is severe with little squirm room or substitutions, and weight loss must be kept up if the low caloric admission is additionally kept up, making it difficult to cling to the long haul. That implies any weight you lost in the initial seven days is probably going to be recovered after you finish," says dr. Youdin. Her primary concern is "restricting protein consumption with juices will bring about a loss of bulk. Losing muscle is synonymous with dropping your metabolic rate or 'digestion,' making weight upkeep progressively difficult," she says.

Chapter 2:
How the sirtfood diet works

Singer Adele has confirmed that she has lost 30kg in just one year. The secret? It's all thanks to the sirtfood diet. The singer herself revealed it through international media, such as the daily mail and the new york post.

The sirtfood diet is not the classic fasting diet: Adele is the living proof of this, given the splendid shape in which was at her appointments with her fans. It is, in fact, a diet that leaves room for both cheese and red wine as well as chocolate, in the right proportions, and of course under the supervision of a specialist doctor, who knows how to evaluate your health and recommend the most suitable diet to lose weight safely.

Many were the media that underlined the substantial weight loss of the singer Adele who admitted, how the decision to lose weight did not depend on the acceptance of herself as much as the difficulty of using her voice to the fullest.

Adele praised the sirtfood diet, which made her lose 30kg without much effort (although in reality, she admitted via Instag that she had never struggled as much in physical activity as when preparing for her tour). She also said that the beauty of sirt foods is that many of them are already on our table every day. They are accessible and can be easily integrated into our diet.

Although being thinner was not her priority (the singer has always had an excellent relationship with her body), she wanted to review her eating habits to get back in shape, but also (or better above all) to feel good about herself.

Furthermore, the sirtfood diet had come back on the news because it was Pippa Middleton's choice to get back into shape quickly before her wedding with the millionaire James Matthews that was celebrated on May 20, 2017.

Pippa Middleton would have tested the concrete benefits of this hunger-free regime by eating the ingredients of the sirtfood diet prepared by nutritionists Aidan Goggins and Glen Matten with gusto. Nothing to do with the Dukan, diet followed by sister Kate before marrying Prince William, one of the many fasting diets that currently exist.

Introduction

The sirtfood diet is a diet named after a molecule in some plant-based foods, called sirtuin activators. Sirtuin activators are a type of protein that helps insulate cells from the effect of ageing, inflammation and several nasty metabolic processes.

Owing to this, sirtuin activators have been associated with longevity, with people who intake high amounts of sirtuin over long periods demonstrably living longer than their peers. There are also numerous other benefits, such as increases in muscle mass and making it easier to burn. The sirtfood diet revolves around, ensuring you keep your sirtuin intake high, promoting weight loss and overall bodily health.

The interesting part of the sirtfood diet is its shift in focus. This isn't a fad diet to lose weight – rather the emphasis is just eating in a healthy and balanced way, with weight loss naturally occurring once your body has been cleansed of your poor eating habits.

There are many foods which contain sirtuin activators, most notably both chocolate and red wine. Of course, the sirtuin diet doesn't claim to be a miracle diet where you can binge on chocolate and wine, if only hey!. You will still need to balance your intake of calories and ensure you receive an even spread of essential food groups too.

The core of the diet consists of healthy sirtuin activator foods, which includes apples, citrus fruits, blueberries, green tea, soy, strawberries, turmeric, olive oil, red onion and kale. There are also a couple of surprises, such as coffee, which is usually reprimanded in most contemporary diets.

However, the problem with fasting diets, as the name implies, is that you have to fast. Fasting feels awful, especially when we are surrounded by other people having regular eating habits. It also puts some social spotlight on your own diet – explaining to your co-workers or your extended family why you are not eating on certain days is bound to generate incredulity and challenges to your diet regime.

Furthermore, even though fasting has numerous associated benefits, there are some downsides too. Fasting is associated with muscle loss, as the body doesn't discriminate between muscle mass and fat tissue when choosing cells to burn for energy.

Fasting also risks malnutrition, simply by not eating enough foods to get essential nutrients. This risk can be somewhat alleviated by taking vitamin supplements and eating nutrient-rich foods, but fasting can also slow and halt the digestive system altogether – preventing the absorption of supplements. These supplements also need dietary fat to be dissolved, which you might also lack if you were to implement a strict fasting.

On top of this, fasting isn't appropriate for a huge range of people. Obviously, you don't want children to fast and potentially inhibit their growth. Likewise, the elderly, the ill and the pregnant are all just too vulnerable to the risks of fasting.

Additionally, there are several psychological detriments to fasting, despite commonly being associated with spiritual revelations. Fasting makes you irritable and causes you to feel slightly on edge – your body is telling you constantly that you need to forage for food, enacting physical processes that affect your mood and emotions.

This is why the authors of the sirtfood diet sought a replacement for fasting diets. Fasting is beneficial for our body, but it just isn't practical for society at large. This is where sirtuin activators and sirtfoods come to the rescue.

Sirtuins were first discovered in 1984 in yeast molecules. Of course, once it became apparent that sirtuin activators affected a variety of factors, such as lifespan and metabolic activity, interest in these proteins blossomed.

Sirtuin activators boost your mitochondria's activity, the part of the biological cell which is responsible for the production of energy. This, in turn, mirrors the energy-boosting effects, which also occur due to exercise and fasting. The sirtfood diet is thought to start a process called adipogenesis, which prevents fat cells from duplicating – which should interest any potential dieter.

The interesting part is that the sirtuin activators influence your genetics. The notion of the 'genetic' lottery is embedded in the public consciousness, but genes are more changeable then you might think. You won't be able to change your eye colour or your height, but you can activate or deactivate specific genes based on environmental factors. This is called epigenetics, and it is a fascinating field of study.

Sirtuin activators cause the sir genes to activate, the before-mentioned 'skinny genes', which in turn increases the release of sirts. Sirts or silent information regulators also help regulate the circadian rhythm, which is your natural body clock and influences sleep patterns.

Sleep is important for many vital biological processes, including those that help regulate blood sugar (which is also important for losing weight). If you find yourself constantly stuck in a state of lag and brain fog, this may be caused by your circadian rhythm being out of sync, which is another way the sirtfood diet can help your body.

Additionally, sirts help contain free radicals. Free radicals are not as awesome as the sound – they are a.w.o.l particles in your body that damage your DNA and speed up the ageing process.

To summarise, the sirtfood diet contains foods which are high in sirtuin activators. Sirtuin activators activate your sir genes or 'skinny genes' which enact beneficial metabolic processes. These processes, which involve molecules, called sirts, causes your body to burn fat, repair bodily cells and combat free radicals.

So, sirtfoods have been hailed as the next dietary wonder – but where is the cold, hard evidence? Well, the evidence for the sirtfood diet comes from multiple sources. To start with, Aidan Goggins and Glen Matten, the originators of the sirtfood diet, performed their own trial at a privately owned fitness centre to test sirtfoods themselves.

At a fitness centre called kx, in Chelsea, London, the two authors of the sirtfood diet made a selection of their clientèle eat a carefully monitored constructed sirtfood diet. What is particularly interesting about the study is that weight wasn't the only variable measured – the researchers also measured body composition and metabolic activity – they were searching for the holistic effect of the diet.

97.5% of people managed to stick to the first-three day fasting period, involving only 1,000 calories. Generally speaking, this is a much higher rate of success than typical fasting diets, where many people have their willpower shattered in just the first few days.

Out of the 40 participants, 39 completed the study. In terms of overall fitness and weight, the individuals in the study were well distributed – 2 were officially obese, 15 fell into the overweight category while 22 had a regular body mass index. There were also 21 women and 18 men – a diet for both the genders! However, with that being said, being members of a fitness centre, the individuals in the study were more likely to exercise more than the standard population – a potential confounding factor.

Participants lost over 7lbs on average in the first week. Every participant experienced an improvement in body composition, even if their gains were not as dramatic as their peers.

There were also numerous reported psychological benefits, although these were not formally quantified. These improvements include an overall sense of feeling and looking better. As a side note, it was also claimed the 40 participants rarely felt hungry, even despite the calorie deficits imposed by the diet.

The most startling result from the sirtfood diet is that muscle mass after the 1-week diet period was either the same as before, or showed slight improvements. Dieting law typically states that when losing fat, muscle is also lost, usually around 20-30% of the total weight loss, you should lose 2-3 lbs of muscle for every 10 lbs lost.

Of course, retaining muscle isn't just better from an overall fitness perspective, but also from an aesthetic view. A common fear, especially in men, is that if they lose weight is that they will look skinny, scrawny and unhealthy. Yet by the retaining the muscle you will gain that toned, slither look that is so fashionable in models.

Another important reason why retaining muscle mass is your resting energy expenditure. Your muscles require energy, even when you are not using them intensely. Owing to this, people who keep skeletal muscle burn more calories than people who don't, even if both people are sedentary. Basically, being muscular allows you to eat more calories and get away with it!

Muscle mass has also been associated with a general decrease in degenerative diseases as you age (such as diabetes and osteoporosis) as well as lower rates of mental health problems (such as depression and excessive anger).

Overall, the clinical trial performed at the kx fitness centre not only supported the notion that the sirtfood diet can aid weight loss and promote holistic body health, but it also leads to the surprising finding that sirtfoods can retain muscle mass.

This is the beauty of the sirtfood diet – it isn't trying to make your eating habits artificial and awkward. It is simply copying the healthiest practices that already exist around the world.

Skeletal muscle is all the muscles you voluntarily control, such as the muscles in your limbs, back, shoulders, and so on. There are two other types: cardiac muscle is what the heart is formed of, while the smooth muscle is your involuntary muscles – which includes muscles around your blood vessels, face and various parts of organs and other tissues.

Skeletal muscle is separated into two different groups, the blandly named type-1 and type-2. Type 1 muscle is effective at continued, sustained activity whereas type-2 muscle is effective at short, intense periods of activity. So, for example, you would predominantly use type-1 muscles for jogging, but type-2 muscles for sprinting.

Sirt-1 protects the type-1 muscles, but not the type-2 muscle, which is still broken down for energy. Therefore, holistic muscle mass drops when fasting, even though type-1 skeletal muscle mass increases.

Sirt-1 also influences how the muscles work. Sirt-1 is produced by the muscle cells, but the ability to produce sirt-1 decreases as the muscle ages. As a result, muscle is harder to build as you age and doesn't grow as fast in response to exercise. A lack of sirt-1 also causes the muscles to become tired quicker and gradually decline over time.

When you start to consider these effects of sirt-1, you can start to form a picture of why fasting helps keep the body supple. Fasting releases sirt-1, which in turn helps skeletal muscle grow and stay in good shape. sirt-1 is also released by consuming sirtuin activators, giving the sirtfood diet its muscle retaining power.

How much sirtfood do you need to eat?

Of course, the sirtfood diet is more than just pumping a bunch of the best sirtfoods into your eating habits. It is a holistic diet with food organised into different meals, each designed to give you the highest sirtuin kick. On top of this, the sirtfood diet isn't exotic.

The main ingredients of the sirtfood diet are common, and you probably use them already, on occasion. The trick is just making sure you are getting enough – the average American only receives 13mg of sirtuins a day – which is five times lower than their Japanese counterparts.

So if sirtuins are so fantastic, why don't we take them as a supplement or pill? The truth is although a pharmaceutical application of sirtuins may be possible in the future, our current understanding of food science and biology is still too limited for this to be effective today.

Understanding how sirtuins are processed and absorbed, which likely depends on other nutrients in food, is crucial to making sirtuins work. At the moment, it is simply easier and more successful to consume sirtuins the natural way, receiving all the extra stuff you need in the sirtfoods themselves.

For example, resveratrol, the sirtuin activator, which is present in certain types of red wine, is known to be absorbed poorly when taken, are a pure substance. When ingested in red-wine, it is in fact absorbed six times better. Simply put, food is complicated and we only understand a few pieces of the puzzle.

Another reason why sirtuins are not taken as a pill or supplement is the fact there are so many of them, all with slightly different effects. Add this to the before-mentioned complexity, and it's better to consume foods where you know you get a natural mix.

Fortunately, this draconian restriction only lasts three days, in which you progress to a four-day stage where you are allotted another 500 calories, and you can replace one of your juices with another sirtfood meal.

Finally, after four more days you progress to phase-2, where you are allowed three full sirtfood meals and one meal juice for another two-weeks. In this period, your focus in on keeping your intake of sirtfoods high and maintaining your weight loss.

You do not need to eat a calorie deficit in phase 2, but nor should you be eating more calories than you need. The sirtfood diet claims that you can maintain weight loss during this period, even without the calorie deficit due to the changes in our body.

After the 14-day maintenance period, you have the freedom to choose your own eating habits. The sirtfood diet isn't a diet for life; rather, it is a temporary change to your eating habits intended to change how your body is processing food.

Therefore whenever you need a fat-burning boost, you can re-implement the three-stage sirtfood dieting process to speed up your weight loss and cleanse your body. Of course, over a longer period, ideally, you should gradually implement more and more sirtfoods into your lifestyle.

You should also make an effort to make sirtfood recipes practical for your family. Batch cooking and freezing will help with the constant demand to cook. Likewise, several recipes are remarkably quick and low-effort and can be used as quick solutions to hungry mouths.

The sirtfood diet was an achievement nourishment system a couple of years and was the dear eating routine with the broadsheet press at the time. If you missed it, the features are that it incorporates red wine, chocolate, and espresso. Far less promoted and eye-catching, (yet similarly uplifting news as we would like to think) is the way that the response to the inquiry, 'would you be able to eat meat on the sirt nourishment diet?', is a resonating, yes.

The eating routine arrangement not just incorporates a decent sound part of the meat; it proceeds to recommend that protein is a basic consideration in a sirtfood-based eating routine to receive the greatest reward.

We're not supporting this as some meat overwhelming eating routine (we despite everything recollect the awful breath from Atkins), it's in reality very veggie-lover cordial and provides food for practically everybody, which is the thing that makes it so reasonable an alternative to us.

So what is the sirtfood diet? Nutritionists created it Aidan Goggins and Glen Matten, following a pilot learn at the elite xk gym, (Daniel Craig, Madonna and an entire host of different celebs are supposedly individuals) where they are the two experts in Sloane Square, London. Members in the preliminary lost 7lbs in the initial seven days, in what the creators call the hyper-achievement to organise. The science behind sirtfoods drops out of an investigation in 2003 which found that a compound found in red wine, expanded the life expectancy of yeast. At last, this prompted the investigations which clarify the medical advantages of red wine, and how (whenever drank reasonably) individuals who drink red wine put on less weight.

A significant part of the science behind the sirtfood diet is like that of 'fasting-diets' which have been well known for as far back as barely any years, whereby our bodies initiate qualities and our fat stockpiling is turned off; our bodies change to endurance mode, thus weight reduction. The negatives to fasting-eats fewer carbs are the unavoidable craving that results, alongside a decrease in vitality, bad-tempered conduct (when you're "hangry"), weariness and muscle misfortune. The sirtfood diet professes to counter those negatives, as it's anything but a quick, so hunger isn't an issue, making it ideal for individuals who need to lead a functioning solid way of life.

Sirtfoods are a (generally newfound) gathering of nourishments that are incredible in actuating the 'sirtuin' qualities in our body, which are the qualities enacted in fasting eats fewer carbs.

Critically for us carnivores, the book proceeds to recommend in the section entitled 'sirtfoods forever' that protein is basic to keep up digestion and decrease the loss of muscle when counting calories. Leucine is an amino corrosive found in protein, which praises and upgrades the activities of sirtfoods. This implies the most ideal approach to eat sirtfoods is by consolidating them with a chicken bosom, steak or another wellspring of leucine, for example, fish or eggs.

Generally, we can thoroughly observe the advantage and intrigue of the sirtfood diet. Like practically any eating regimen plan, it tends to be a faff getting every one of the fixings, and the 'sirtfood green juice', which shapes a centrepiece of the initial 14 days of the arrangement, is a torment to make and is costly, yet it shows improvement over you'd anticipate. We just trialled a couple of days of the arrangement and keeping in mind that there was perceptible weight reduction, the genuine advantage of the book is the reasonable Directions ology of bringing sirtfoods into your regular dinner arranging.

Chapter 3:
How to follow the sirt food diet

Phase 1 of the diet is the one that produces the greatest results. Over the course of seven days, you will follow simple directions to lose 3.5kg. Following, you will find a step-by-step guide, complete with menus and recipes.

During the first three days, the intake of calories will have to be limited to 1,000 per day at most. You can have three green juices and a solid meal, all based on sirt foods. From day 4 to 7, the daily calories will become fifteen hundred. Every day you will eat two green juices and two solid sirt meals. By the end of the seven days, you should have lost, on average, 3.5kg.

Despite the reduction in calories, the participants do not feel hungry, and the calorie limit is an indication rather than a goal. Even in the most intensive phase, calorie restriction is not as drastic as in many other regimes. Sirt foods have a naturally satiating effect so that many of you will feel pleasantly full and satisfied.

Phase 2 is the maintenance phase and lasts 14 days: during this period, although the main objective is not the reduction of calories, you will consolidate weight loss and continue to lose weight. The secret to succeeding at this stage lies in continuing to eat sirt foods in abundance; following the prog that we will provide you with relative recipes will facilitate you. During those two weeks, you will consume three balanced and rich sirt foods per day and a green sirt juice.

Phase 1

Monday: 3 green juices | breakfast: water + tea or espresso + a cup of green juice; | lunch: green juice | snack: a square of dark chocolate | dinner: sirt meal | after dinner: a square of dark chocolate.

Drink the juices at three distinct times of the day (for example, in the morning as soon as you wake up, mid-morning and mid-afternoon) and choose the normal or vegan dish: pan-fried oriental prawns with buckwheat spaghetti or miso and tofu with sesame glaze and sautéed vegetables (vegan dish).

Tuesday: 3 green juices | breakfast: water + tea or espresso + a cup of green juice | lunch: 2 green juices | before dinner snack: a square of dark chocolate | dinner: sirt meal | after dinner: a square of dark chocolate.

Welcome to day 2 of the sirtfood diet. The formula is identical to that of the first day, and the only thing that changes is the solid meal. Today you will also have dark chocolate, and the same goes for tomorrow. This food is so wonderful that we don't need an excuse to eat it.

To earn the title of a "sirt food", chocolate must be at least 85% cocoa, and even among the various types of chocolate with this percentage, not all of them are the same. Often this product is treated with an alkalising agent (this is the so-called "dutch process") to reduce its acidity and give it a darker colour. Unfortunately, this process greatly reduces the flavonoids activating sirtuins, compromising their health benefits. Lindt excellence 85% chocolate, is not subjected to the dutch process and is therefore often recommended.

On day 2, capers are also included in the menu. Despite what many may think, they are not fruits, but buds that grow in Mediterranean countries and are picked by hand. They are fantastic sirt foods because they are very rich in the nutrients kaempferol and quercetin. From the point of view of flavour, they are tiny concentrates of taste. If you've never used them, don't feel intimidated. You will see, they will taste amazingly if combined with the right ingredients, and they will give an unmistakable and inimitable aroma to your dishes.

On the second day, you will intake 3 green sirt juices and 1 solid meal (normal or vegan).

Drink the juices at three distinct times of the day (for example, when you wake up in the morning, mid-morning and mid-afternoon) and choose either the normal or the vegan dish: turkey escalope with capers, parsley, and sage on spiced cauliflower couscous or curly kale and red onion dahl with buckwheat (vegan dish).

Wednesday: 3 green juices | breakfast: water + tea or espresso + a cup of green juice | lunch: 2 green juices | before dinner snack: a square of dark chocolate | dinner: sirt meal | after dinner: a square of dark chocolate.

You are now on the third day, and even if the format is once again identical to that of days 1 and 2, so the time has come to flavour everything with a fundamental ingredient. For thousands of years, chilli has been a fundamental element of the gastronomic experiences of the whole world.

If you are not a big expert of chilli, we recommend the bird's eye (sometimes called Thai chilli) because it is the best for sirtuins.

This is the last day you will consume three green juices a day; tomorrow, you will switch to two. We, therefore, take this opportunity to browse other drinks that you can have during the diet. We all know that green tea is good for health, and water is naturally very good, but what about coffee? More than half of people drink at least one coffee a day, but always with a trace of guilt because some say that it is a vice and an unhealthy habit. This is untrue; studies show that coffee is a real treasure trove of beneficial plant substances. That's why coffee drinkers run the least risk of getting diabetes, certain forms of cancer, and neurodegenerative diseases. Furthermore, not only is coffee, not a toxin, it protects the liver and makes it even healthier!

On the third day, you will intake 3 green sirt juices and 1 solid meal (normal or vegan, see below).

Drink the juices at three distinct times of the day (for example, in the morning as soon as you wake up, mid-morning and mid-afternoon) and choose the normal or vegan dish: aromatic chicken breast with kale, red onion, tomato sauce, and chilli or baked tofu with harissa on spiced cauliflower couscous (vegan dish).

Thursday: 3 green juices | breakfast: water + tea or espresso + a cup of green juice | lunch: sirt food | snack: 1 green juice before dinner | dinner: sirt food

The fourth day of the sirtfood diet has arrived, and you are halfway through your journey to a leaner and healthier body. The big change from the previous three days is that you will only drink two juices instead of three and that you will have two solid meals instead of one. This means that on the fourth day and the upcoming ones, you will have two green juices and two solid meals, all delicious and rich in sirt foods. The inclusion of Medjool dates in a list of foods that promote weight loss and good health may seem surprising. Especially when you think they contain 66% sugar.

Sugar has no stimulating properties towards sirtuins. On the contrary, it has well-known links with obesity, heart disease, and diabetes; in short, just at the antipodes of the objectives, we aim to. But industrially refined and processed sugar is very different from the sugar present in a food that also contains sirtuin-activating polyphenols: the Medjool dates. Unlike regular sugar, these dates, consumed in moderation, do not increase the level of glucose in the blood.

Today we will also integrate chicory into meals. Like with onion, red chicory is better in this case too, but endive, its close relative, is also a sirt food. If you are looking for ideas on the use of these salads, combine them with other varieties and season them with olive oil: they will give a pungent flavour to milder leaves.

On the fourth day, you will intake: 2 green sirt juices, 2 solid meals (normal or vegan) drink the juices at different times of the day (for example the first in the morning as soon as you wake up or in the middle of the morning, the second in the middle of the afternoon) and choose the normal or vegan dishes: muesli sirt, pan-fried salmon fillet with caramelised chicory, rocket salad, and celery leaves or muesli sirt and Tuscan stewed beans (vegan dish).

Friday: 2 green juices | breakfast: water + tea or espresso + a cup of green juice | lunch: sirt food | snack: a green juice before dinner | dinner: sirt food

You have reached the fifth day, and the time has come to add fruits. Due to its high sugar content, fruits have been the subject of bad publicity. This does not apply to berries. Strawberries have a very low sugar content: one tsp per 100 gs. They also have an excellent effect on how the body processes simple sugars.

Scientists have found that if we add strawberries to simple sugars, this causes a reduction in insulin demand, and therefore transforms food into a machine that releases energy for a long time. Strawberries are, therefore, a perfect element in diets that will help you lose weight and get back in shape. They are also delicious and extremely versatile, as you will discover in the sirt version of the fresh and light middle eastern tabbouleh.

Miso, made from fermented soy, is a traditional Japanese dish. Miso contains a strong umami taste, a real explosion for the taste buds. In our modern society, we know better monosodium glutamate, artificially created to reproduce the same flavour. Needless to say, it is far preferable to derive that magical umami flavour from traditional and natural food, full of beneficial substances. It is found in the form of a paste in all good supermarkets and healthy food stores and should be present in every kitchen to give a touch of taste to many different dishes.

Since umami flavours enhance each other, miso is perfectly associated with other tasty/umami foods, especially when it comes to cooked proteins, as you will discover today in the delicious, fast and easy dishes you will eat.

On the fifth day, you will intake 2 green sirt juices and 2 solid meals (normal or vegan).

Drink the juices at different times of the day (for example the first in the morning as soon as you wake up or in the middle of the morning, the second in the middle of the afternoon) and choose the normal or vegan dishes.

Saturday: 2 green juices | breakfast: water + tea or espresso + a cup of green juice | lunch: sirt food | snack: a green juice before dinner | dinner: sirt food

There are no sirt foods better than olive oil and red wine. Virgin olive oil is obtained from the fruit only by mechanical means, in conditions that do not deteriorate it, so that you can be sure of its quality and polyphenol content. "extra virgin" oil is that of the first pressing ("virgin" is the result of the second) and therefore has more flavour and better quality: this is what we strongly recommend you to use when cooking.

No sirt menu would be complete without red wine, one of the cornerstones of the diet. It contains the activators of resveratrol and piceatannol sirtuins, which probably explain the longevity and slenderness associated with the traditional french way of life, and which are at the origin of the enthusiasm unleashed by sirt foods.

Of course, wine contains alcohol, so it should be consumed in moderation. Fortunately, resveratrol can withstand heat well, and therefore can be used in the kitchen. Pinot noir is many people's favourite grape variety because it contains much more resveratrol than most of the others.

On the sixth day, you will assume 2 green sirt juices and 2 solid meals (normal or vegan).

Drink the juices at different times of the day (for example, the first in the morning as soon as you wake up or in the middle of the morning, the second in the middle of the afternoon) and choose the normal or vegan dishes: super sirt salad and grilled beef fillet with red wine sauce, onion rings, garlic curly kale and roasted potatoes with aromatic herbs or super lentil sirt salad (vegan dish) and mole sauce of red beans with roasted potato (vegan dish).

Sunday: 2 green juices | breakfast: a bowl of sirt muesli + a cup of green juice | lunch: sirt food | snack: a cup of green juice | dinner: sirt food

The seventh day is the last of phase 1 of the diet. Instead of considering it as an end, see it as a beginning, because you are about to embark on a new life, in which sirt foods will play a central role in your nutrition. Today's menu is a perfect example of how easy it is to integrate them in abundance into your daily diet. Just take your favourite dishes and, with a pinch of creativity, you will turn them into a sirt banquet.

Walnuts are excellent sirt food because they contradict current opinions. They have high-fat content and many calories, yet it has been shown that they contribute to reducing weight and metabolic diseases, all thanks to the activation of sirtuins. They are also a versatile ingredient, excellent in baked dishes, in salads and as a snack, alone.

Pesto is becoming an irreplaceable ingredient in the kitchen because it is tasty and allows you to give personality to even the simplest dishes. The traditional one is made with basil and pine nuts, but you can try an alternative one with parsley and walnuts. The result is delicious and rich in sirt foods.

We can apply the same reasoning to an easy-to-prepare dish, such as an omelette. The dish has to be the typical recipe appreciated by the whole family, and simple to transform into a sirt dish with a few little tricks. In our recipe, we use bacon. Why? Simply because it fits perfectly. The sirtfood diet tells us what to include, not what to exclude, and this allows us to change our long-term eating habits. After all, isn't that the secret to not getting back the lost pounds and staying healthy?

On the seventh day, you will assume 2 green sirt juices; 2 solid meals (normal or vegan).

Drink the juices at different times of the day (for example the first in the morning as soon as you wake up or in the middle of the morning, the second in the middle of the afternoon) and choose the normal or vegan dishes.

During the second phase, there are no calorie restrictions but indications on which sirt foods must be eaten to consolidate weight loss and not run the risk of getting the lost kilos back.

The procedure of the sirtfood diet

The sirt food diet consists of three phases: in phase one, the body is relieved as with a gentle fast. In the second phase, you lose pounds; in the third phase, you keep the desired weight.

Sometimes two phases are spoken of, in which case the first phase consists of phase 1 and 2.

You can repeat these three phases as often as you want to lose weight. However, we recommend that you continue to "sirtify" your diet after these phases are complete by regularly including sirt foods in your meals. We also recommend that you continue drinking green juice or smoothies every day.

The 3 phases of the sirtfood diet:

- Phase 1: the first phase is the reprogramming of the metabolism to "lean". This works, for example, with sirtuin-rich green juices that detoxify the body. It lasts for three days. This means 1,000 calories per day in the form of 3 juices and 1 main meal.

- Phase 2: the calorie intake is increased to 1,500 calories. It lasts for four days. There are now 2 green juices and 2 main meals per day.

- Phase 3: serves to stabilise the new weight. In the third or "maintenance" phase, everything is allowed as long as you have as many sirt foods on the menu as possible and eat about 1800 calories. It lasts for two weeks. There are 1 green juice and 3 main meals per day.

Meal plan for three weeks

Phase 1, day 1-3:

In the first three days, you only consume 1,000kcal at a time. To be consumed:

• 3x green sirtfood juice • 1x main meal

Phase 2, day 4-7:

In the next four days, you will reach 1.500kcal. This is achieved by

• 2x green sirtfood juice • 2x main meal

During the introductory phase, you should drink water, green tea and black coffee.

Phase 3, day 8-21:

The second phase then lasts 14 days. There is also a fixed plan here, based on which there are:

• 1x green sirtfood juice • 3x main meal • 1-2x snacks

You should drink the juice first, about 30 minutes before breakfast. The dinner should be taken until 7 pm if possible. You should drink water, green tea or black coffee. Black or white tea is also fine. Red wine is also allowed, but not more than two to three glasses per week, otherwise the fat will be stored again.

Day 1

-3x green sirtfood juice

-1x main meal

Day 2

-3x green sirtfood juice

-1x main meal

Day 3

-3x green sirtfood juice

-1x main meal

Day 4

-2x green sirtfood juice

-2x main meal

Day 5

-2x green sirtfood juice

-2x main meal

Day 6

-2x green sirtfood juice

-2x main meal

Day 7

-2x green sirtfood juice

-2x main meal

Day 8

-1x green sirtfood juice

-3x main meal

Day 9

-1x green sirtfood juice

-3x main meal

Day 10

-1x green sirtfood juice

-3x main meal

Day 11

-1x green sirtfood juice

-3x main meal

Day 12

-1x green sirtfood juice

-3x main meal

Day 13

-1x green sirtfood juice

-3x main meal

Day 14

-1x green sirtfood juice

-3x main meal

Day 15

-1x green sirtfood juice

-3x main meal

Day 16

-1x green sirtfood juice

-3x main meal

Day 17

-1x green sirtfood juice

-3x main meal

Day 18

-1x green sirtfood juice

-3x main meal

Day 19

-1x green sirtfood juice

-3x main meal

Day 20

-1x green sirtfood juice

-3x main meal

Day 21

-1x green sirtfood juice

-3x main meal

Expectations for phase 1

In the first seven days of the diet, you should anticipate losing up to 7 lbs. The wording of this sentence is important – you may lose 7 lbs, but many people don't see such dramatic changes.

Bear in mind that the sirtfood diet may also result in a gain in muscle mass, another reason why the 7 lbs loss may not be achieved. Instead of the precise weight value, it's better to look for signs that your body is changing. Do your clothes fit better? Do you feel better? Has your skin improved?

Looking for other signs of the diet is also important because the sirtfood diet isn't just a weight loss scheme – it is intended to promote overall body health, so you should anticipate overall improvements. The authors of the sirtfood diet even go so far as to suggest that you can purchase some basic health measurement tools from your local pharmacies, such as a blood pressure monitor or blood sugar monitor to check for changes.

Finally, you need to change your outlook. The sirtfood diet is intended to replace your normal eating habits eventually, and so you need to go into the diet with a willingness and adaptivity to generate a long-term change.

It is recommended that you space your three juices out between the day, instead of consuming them in rapid succession. You should avoid drinking any of the juices any hour before or after your main meal.

It is also suggested that you should also not consume any of your juices, or your main meal, after 7 pm. This is advised due to our natural circadian rhythms (or our 'body clock') and how they affect our body. Generally speaking, our body wants to prepare and burn energy in the morning, while store and retain energy during the evening. Therefore if you eat later at night, you have a higher chance of the energy in your food being stored as fat.

In fact, some evidence also supports the idea that sirtuins can enhance and support the circadian rhythm, increasing the amount of energy you burn in the morning.

On top of this, it is also advised that you don't force yourself to eat your meal or consume your juices if you feel too full. Surprisingly, although you are at a notable calorie deficit during the first few days, many people report that they don't feel hungry. In fact, the contrast is true, with people often claiming they are completely stuffed. Owing to this, if you can't consume all your intake of the first few days, don't worry.

You should also feel free to drink non-calorie fluids. While this technically does include calorie-free fizzy drinks, the authors of the diet promote green tea, black coffee and of course, water, as good choices. One surprising finding is that small doses of lemon juice can prove helpful in increasing sirtuin absorption, so consider add a dash to your water or green tea.

Note that only black coffee is heartily recommended, with milk, sugar and sweeteners diminishing the sirtuin absorption and interfering with the calorie count. Another caveat is that you shouldn't change your coffee consumption too much from your regular habits. A sudden drop in consumption will make you feel awful; a sharp increase will make you feel jittery. Change your coffee habits gradually.

Day-by-day breakdown

Day 1, 2 & 3 you should be aware of the formula by now – three green juices taken in the morning, midday and evening with a main meal in between. You can select any of the main meals covered in the recipe section.

Additionally, you can also have 20g of dark chocolate, as long as the chocolate is at least 85% cocoa solids. There's also a process called dutch processing which is applied to chocolate that diminishes the nutritional value. As a result, you should try to avoid certain brands that use dutch processing by choosing alternative brands.

Day 4, 5, 6 & 7. Your calorie count gets increased to 1,500, and you drop one of the green juices for a second main meal. You also, unfortunately, drop the chocolate. Ensure that you are not repetitive with your selection of meals – you need variety and you shouldn't have needed to repeat a meal, as of yet.

How to jumpstart your sirtfood diet?

Fat burning, increasing muscles, and better cellular fitness – these are the guaranteed results of the sirtfood diet.

Being healthy and losing weight is an everyday choice. You have to take those first baby steps and see how it can change you and your life.

If you want to reap the fantastic results of sirtfoods, here are some suggested ways to jumpstart your diet:

Safety first - before starting any particular diet or regimen, consult your healthcare provider, especially if you have existing illnesses. This will ensure that the diet will not sabotage any medications that you might be taking or harm your health. Do not worry; the sirtfood diet is safe.

Knowledge is power - this diet is still brand new, but there is still a good amount of information available and more upcoming since this diet is fast gaining popularity. Also, you can search the internet for recipes, food alternatives, nutrient content and more.

Follow the guidelines - sirtfood is guaranteed to bring results, if and only if you carefully follow the diet guide and suggested food.

Help yourself - aside from following what is allowed in the food prog; you can start by eliminating processed and starchy food from your normal diet. Stop eating junk! This will fast track the result of sirtfood diet.

Start a physical activity - sirtfood diet can indeed burn those fats and build muscle, but I recommend that you start adding physical activities to your daily routine. A 30-minute walk a day would do wonders to your body and will also fast track the results. Also, there are many wonderful effects when exercising like preventing and combating health conditions, helping improve your mood, promoting better sleep, burning calories, giving you an energy boost and more.

Hit the supermarket - the sirtfood diet depends on certain foods. These foods were chosen because of their sirtuin-triggering ability. So if you do not follow the list, well, you won't see results. Do not worry, because I will be providing a list of suggested foods; plus there are no overly expensive type of foods, and you can find it readily available almost anywhere (you might even already have some lurking in your fridge).

Be ready with the initial "restrictions" - of course, if you want to see different results, you have to "sacrifice" a little to achieve the full benefits of the sirtfood diet. But don't worry, the first three days are only the hardest ones for this diet since there will be calorie restrictions involved, but rest assured that it will become easier each day. Although for others who tried the diet, the restrictions set was not that hard for them, the reason is careful planning of meals. You will not go hungry with this diet if you choose wisely.

Involve a diet partner - this diet could also greatly benefit your family, partner or friends (not only for overweight individuals), plus it is easier when you have an accountability partner to remind you, share recipes with or even cook dishes with.

Document your progress - you can start by taking "before" pictures and take necessary body measurements. You could also keep a food diary so that you can watch your food intake. Observe the changes in your body with each week or phase. You can also have a set of goals to push you further to continue with the diet.

Be kind to yourself - do not set too high expectations. Yes, some can easily lose 7lbs in a week, but remember that our bodies are not all the same; and of course, your level of commitment will also count. Other variables could be adding an exercise regimen in the diet plan, which could make the losing weight process faster.

Chapter 4:
What's a "skinny gene"?

The skinny gene-diet is not difficult to follow and is divided into two phases. The first phase lasts 7 days and is more restrictive and difficult, especially for the first 3 days. To be able to lose 3 kg per week as promised by this diet, it is advisable, initially, not to exceed 1,000 calories per day during the first 3 days, drinking 3 green juices based on sirtuin-rich foods and eating only one solid meal of your choice, prepared using the ingredients indicated above.

From the 4th to the 7th day, instead, you can ingest 1,500 calories per day by consuming three green juices and two solid meals composed of foods rich in sirtuins.

The sirtfood diet also called the skinny gene-diet, is the result of the studies of the two nutritionists Aidan Goggins and Glenn Matten. Their food prog, published in a volume that explains its principles and functioning, has attracted the attention of VIPs and athletes. Its effectiveness is based on the consumption of foods that stimulate sirtuins. As the creators of the diet of the moment explain, it is a family of genes present in each of us. They affect the ability to burn fat in addition to mood and the mechanisms that regulate longevity. It is no coincidence that they are also called "super metabolic regulators." Recent studies have shown that several foods can stimulate sirtuins. Their consumption would, therefore, allow them to activate the metabolism and lose weight without having to undergo extreme diets.

What makes the sirtfood diet different from the others is its "inclusion" philosophy. In fact, it is not based on the total or partial exclusion of some foods from your diet. Rather, it suggests which foods should be added to lose weight more easily. In this way, you will no longer have to undergo excessive deprivation or exhausting willpower. And you won't have to resort to expensive supplements or products with mysterious components. By eating a balanced diet and supporting it, if desired, with proper physical activity, according to the two nutritionists, you can lose about 3.5kg in a week.

Sirt foods are particularly rich in special nutrients, capable of activating the same genes of thinness stimulated by fasting. These genes are sirtuins. They became famous thanks to an important study conducted in 2003, during which scientists analysed a particular substance, resveratrol, present in the peel of black grapes, red wine, and yeast, which would produce the same effects of calorie restriction without need to decrease your daily calories intake. Later, researchers found that other substances in red wine had a similar effect, which would explain the benefits of consuming this drink and why those who consume it get less fat.

This naturally stimulated the search for other foods containing a high concentration of these nutrients, capable of producing such a beneficial effect on the body, and studies gradually discovered several. If some are almost unknown, such as lovage, an herb that is by now very little used in cooking, the great majority is represented by well-known and widely used foods, such as extra virgin olive oil, red onions, parsley, chilli, kale, strawberries, capers, tofu, cocoa, green tea, and even coffee.

After the discovery in 2003, the enthusiasm for the benefits of sort's food skyrocketed. Studies revealed that these foods don't just mimic the effects of calorie restriction. They also act as super regulators of the entire metabolism: they burn fat, increase muscle mass, and improve the health of our cells. The world of medical research was close to the most important nutritional discovery of the century. Unfortunately, a mistake was made: the pharmaceutical industry invested hundreds of millions of pounds in an attempt to turn sirt foods into a sort of miracle pill, and the diet took a back seat. The sirtfood diet, however, does not share this pharmaceutical approach, which seeks (so far without result) to concentrate the benefits of these complex nutrients of plant origin into a single drug. Instead of waiting for the pharmaceutical industry to transform the nutrients of the foods we eat into a miraculous product (which may not work anyway), the sirtfood diet consists of eating these substances in their natural form that of food, to take full advantage of them. This is the basis of the pilot experiment of the sirtfood diet, with which the creators intended to create a diet containing the richest sources of sirt foods and observe their effects.

During their studies, Glen Matten and Aidan Goggins discovered that the best sirt foods are consumed regularly by populations who boast the lowest incidence of diseases and obesity in the world.

The Kuna Indians, in the American continent, seem immune from hypertension and with very low levels of obesity, diabetes, cancer, and early death thanks to the intake of cocoa, excellent sirt food. In Okinawa, Japan, sirt food, dry physique, and longevity go hand in hand. In India, the passion for spicy foods, especially turmeric, gives good results in the fight against cancer. And in the traditional Mediterranean diet, which the rest of the western world envies, obesity is contained, and chronic diseases are the exception, not the norm. extra virgin olive oil, wild green leafy vegetables, dried fruit, berries, red wine, dates, and aromatic herbs are all effective sirt foods, and they are all present in the Mediterranean diet. The scientific world has had to surrender to the evidence: it seems that the Mediterranean diet is more effective than reducing calories to lose weight and more effective than drugs to eliminate diseases.

Although sirt foods are not a mainstay of nutrition in most of the western world today, the situation was quite different in the past. They were a basic element, and if many have become rare and others have even disappeared, it is definitely possible to reverse the course of this.

The good news is that you don't have to be a top athlete, and not even sporty, to enjoy the same benefits. We took advantage of everything we learned about sirt foods thanks to the pilot study by kx and the work done with sportsmen, and we adapted it to create a diet suitable for anyone who wants to lose weight while improving health.

It is not necessary to practice unsustainable fasting or to undergo endless sessions in the gym (although, of course, practising a little physical activity would be good for you). It is not an expensive diet, nor will it waste your time, and all the foods recommended in the diet are readily available. The only accessory you will need is an extractor or centrifuge. Unlike other diets, which tell you what to eliminate, this diet tells you what to eat.

Generally, you can eat foods that are high in protein and low in fat. Among the meat-based recipes, you can choose, for example, chicken with red onion and black cabbage, turkey with cauliflower couscous, turkey escalope with capers and parsley. For fish dishes, sautéed salmon fillet, sautéed prawns, or baked marinated cod are fine.

Recipes of side dishes, light and tasty, can be prepared with beans, lentils, aubergines cut into wedges, and cooked in the oven, Walldorf salad, or red onions. And as for dessert, you can eat delicious and healthy strawberries, with a very high content of sirtuins. Plus, remember that 15-20g of dark chocolate are allowed every day.

The green juice is an important part of the diet, because it has the ability to cleanse and detoxify, and will be the protagonist in the first week of the sirt prog.

Sirt foods are particularly rich in special nutrients of plant origin recently discovered, which, stimulated by fasting, activate the genes of thinness.

The foods suggested in the sirtfood diet are fresh, genuine and easily available, such as extra virgin olive oil, dark chocolate, citrus fruits, strawberries, apples, cabbage, celery, spinach, buckwheat, blueberries, nuts, soya beans, rocket salad, red onion, coffee, green tea**, red wine, chilli pepper***, tofu, turmeric, and dates.

In addition, combined with each other or with other foods, they allow you to create very tasty dishes.

Sirtuins filled ingredients

Cocoa

Yes, to chocolate, but not any type! It must be dark chocolate and present at least 85% of cocoa. Useful above all to appease hunger, therefore mostly used as a snack.

Lindt excellence 85%, which retains a good percentage of flavonoids, and Rowntree's cocoa powder are the most highly recommended.

Chilli pepper***

To make your dishes spicier, use bird's eye chilli (also called Thai chilli), very rich in sirtuin. You can use it at least three times a week.

Warning! Compared to normal chilli, the bird's eye is much spicier; to get used to it, in the beginning, use only half of what is indicated in the recipe, eliminating the seeds, which are very spicy.

Coffee

You can drink 3-4 cups of coffee a day being careful not to overdo it with sugar, and avoid adding milk.

Green tea**

Known because it is so good for our body, green tea contributes to the loss of fat, preserving your muscles. Choose the matcha variety and drink it with the addition of a little lemon juice, which increases the absorption of the nourishing activators of sirtuins.

Red wine

The research that gave rise to the sirtfood diet started with red wine. The first sirt slimming element discovered, in fact, is resveratrol, present in black grape's skin and red wine. It appears that this nutrient attacks fat cells. In addition, red wine contains piceatannol, associated with longevity.

Kale

Kale is a suitable food for every diet. It is cheap and easy to find. It contains in large quantities two nutrients that activate sirtuins: kaempferol and quercetin, which act in synergy to prevent the formation of fat.

Buckwheat

This "pseudo-cereal" is very popular in Japan and is a nutritious and highly satiating food, properties on which this type of nutrition focuses. So yes, to seeds, flakes, and buckwheat pasta.

Celery

The nutritive parts of celery, used for millennia, also as a medicinal plant, are the heart and the leaves: here, in fact, the activators of the sirtuins are contained, which are apigenin and luteolin. A tip: if you can, choose the green one instead of the white one.

Medjoul dates

Although dates are composed of 66% sugar, they also contain "good" polyphenols that activate sirtuins. So, unlike normal sugars, date nutrients do not increase the amount of glucose in the blood, but their consumption seems instead associated with a lower incidence of diabetes and heart disease. However, always remember to eat them in moderation!

Capers

The caper plant is widespread in Mediterranean countries, and its fruits are highly appreciated for their "concentrate of taste" capable of reviving even the most anonymous dishes. Taste aside, capers are also very rich in active-sirtuin nutrients, such as kaempferol and quercetin.

Extra virgin olive oil

Good and healthy, the extra virgin olive oil, obtained from the first pressing of the olives, is a perfect seasoning and tastes very good both on vegetables and on bread! Rich in polyphenols, vitamin-e and "good" fatty acids, it will be your heart and youth's best friend, thanks to its antioxidant properties.

Rocket salad

Arugula is a vegetable rich in nutrients that activate the metabolism, such as quercetin and kaempferol. Its peppery and decisive flavour can embellish many recipes, and it especially goes with olive oil.

A curiosity: they began to cultivate it for the first time in ancient Rome, where it seems it was very appreciated for its aphrodisiac qualities.

Parsley

It is a basic ingredient to enrich practically any dish and a lot of sauces. It tastes fresh and is used to relieve itching and toothache. The sirtfood diet appreciates it above all because it is one of the foods with the highest concentration of apigenin, an activator of sirtuins.

Red chicory

It can be consumed within this diet in large quantities, both alone and accompanied by other sirt foods. A greedy idea? Caramelized red chicory salad with celery leaves.

Soy

In addition to its beneficial properties, associated with the activating action of daidzein and formononetin, soy has an unmistakable flavour that makes every dish tastier.

Soy sauce, soy yoghurt, and miso, a traditional Japanese dish based on salt-fermented soybeans, are all amazing. Red (saltier) and brown miso, are the most suitable qualities to prepare sirt recipes

Red onion

Tasty and rich in quercetin, which activates the metabolism. It is important to peel it and consume it raw to keep the nutrients active so that they can act better on sirtuins.

Strawberries

They have few sugars, are delicious and will also make you lose weight because they are the main source of fisetin, a sirtuin activator.

Walnuts

They are rich in fats and very caloric, yet, according to sirt nutritionists, this food should promote weight loss by also fighting metabolic diseases. In addition, walnuts contain a lot of minerals, which are extremely useful for the body, such as magnesium, zinc, copper, calcium, and iron. An idea for a first course? Try an alternative pesto with walnuts and parsley.

Supplements

In the presence of food deficiencies, it may be appropriate to restore the body's balance by providing it with an extra dose of those nutrients that are missing or are in short supply in our everyday diet. However, remember that supplements shouldn't be eaten "for fun", so it is always advisable to seek medical advice before taking any product, even if it is as natural as it comes.

What does the sirtfood diet include?

Stage 1 of the sirtfood diet is the hyper-achievement stage, a 7-day plan demonstrated to help lose 7lbs. During the initial three days, calorie admission is confined to 1,000 calories for every day, comprising of three sirtfood green juices, in addition to one full dinner rich in sirtfoods. On days four to seven, calorie consumption increments to 1,500 calories, involving two sirtfood-rich green juices and two sirtfood-rich suppers.

Stage 2 is a 14-day upkeep stage, where weight loss proceeds consistently. It's tied in with pressing the diet brimming with an abundance of sirtfoods which is accomplished by eating three adjusted sirtfood-rich dinners day by day, alongside a 'support' sirtfood green juice.

In our sirtfood diet, preliminary members lost a great 7lbs over the underlying 7 days remembering increments for muscle and muscle work. This emotional impact on fat-consuming, while advancing muscle, is one reason that our sirtfood-based diet has gotten so mainstream with anybody needing to get slender and fit as a fiddle, much the same as the world-class competitors and models who have supported along these lines of eating. Alongside fat consuming, sirtfoods additionally have the extraordinary capacity to normally satisfy hunger making them the ideal answer for accomplishing a sound weight and continuing it long haul.

Be that as it may, to consider it absolutely as a weight loss diet is to overlook the main issue. This is a diet that has as a lot to do with health as waistlines. Expanded vitality, more clear skin, feeling alarm progressively, and better rest is the charming 'symptoms' from along these lines of eating. Now and again, the advantages are much progressively exceptional, remembering situations where following the diet for the more drawn out term has turned around metabolic ailments. Such is their wellbeing improving impacts that reviews demonstrate them to be all the more dominant then physician endorsed medicates in forestalling constant malady, with benefits in diabetes, coronary illness and Alzheimer's to give some examples. It's no big surprise that it is entrenched that the way of life eating the most sirtfoods have been the least fatty and most beneficial on the planet.

The primary concern is clear: if you need to accomplish a progressively fiery, less fatty and more advantageous body, and establish the frameworks for lifelong wellbeing and protection from sickness, then the sirtfood diet is for you.

Here at the international food information council foundation, we ramble about trend diets. For the most part, we're exposing them and advancing a fair eating arrangement with space for guilty pleasures and festivities. Now and then the diets we talk about depend on some strong sustenance rules, and others we can't accept truly exist. This next diet we're going to discuss falls into the last class. The most recent on the diet scene is the sirtfood diet, and we're here to disclose to you why you needn't bother with that sort of limitation in your life: it's not science-based or practical.

Chapter 5:
Cancer preventing superfoods

The best thing about this diet is that you are not always forced to starve yourself. Phase 1 and phase 2 can be repeated from time to time to lose fat if necessary. For someone, it might be essential to repeat them every three months, while for someone other people, it will be enough to repeat it once a year. The rest of the time, you are free to live your life, skinnier, and healthier than before, continuing to enjoy the benefits of a diet rich in sirt foods. In fact, these foods have a universal application and can be incorporated in any type of dietary regime: vegan, gluten-free, low in carbohydrates, intermittent fasting, and so on. Incorporating significant quantities of sirt foods will enhance the weight loss and health benefits of all those approaches.

The secret of success is to achieve results that will last a lifetime, and the sirtfood diet is truly exceptional in that sense. When you will have assimilated the cornerstones of a balanced diet and the correct use of supplements, and you have discovered the practical tips to consume even more sirt foods, you will be ready to benefit from them for the rest of your life.

Here is a list of the benefits of the sirtfood diet: promotes fat loss, not muscle loss; you will not regain weight after the end of the diet; you will look better; you will feel better, and you will have more energy; you will avoid fasting and feeling hungry; you will not have to undergo exhausting physical exercises; this diet promotes a longer, healthier life and keeps diseases away.

The benefits of the sirtfood diet are many, besides obviously that of slimming. Activators of sirtuins would lead to a noticeable muscle building, decreased appetite, and improved memory. In addition, the sirtfood diet normalizes the level of sugar in the blood and is able to cleanse the cells from the accumulation of harmful free radicals.

The sirtfood diet depends on a newfound gathering of nourishments called sirtfoods. These miracle nourishments can initiate an amazing reusing process in the body that gets out cell waste and consumes fat. They do this by enacting our sirtuin qualities – otherwise called our "thin" qualities. These are similar qualities that are actuated by exercise and fasting.

Top sirtfoods incorporate kale, rocket, parsley, red onions, strawberries, pecans, additional virgin olive oil, cocoa, curry flavours, green tea and espresso (truly, espresso!). As opposed to past advanced diets where the emphasis is on removing nourishments, with sirtfoods, the advantages are harvested through eating.

Chapter 6:
Breakfast

Cranberry quinoa breakfast

Preparation time: 10 minutes| Cooking time: 20 minutes| Servings: 2

Ingredients:

½ cup quinoa

1 cup milk

2-3 tbsp honey, optional

1 tsp cinnamon

½ tsp vanilla

1 tsp ground flaxseed

2 tbsp walnuts or almonds, chopped

2 tbsp dried cranberries

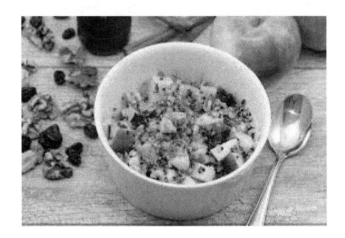

Directions:

Rinse quinoa and drain.

Combine milk, quinoa and flaxseed into a saucepan.

Bring to a boil, add in cinnamon and vanilla and simmer for about 15 minutes.

When done, place a portion of the quinoa into a bowl, drizzle with honey, and top with cranberries and crushed walnuts.

Green omelet

Preparation time: 10 minutes| Cooking time: 30 minutes| Servings: 2

Ingredients:

2 large eggs, at room temperature

1 shallot, peeled and chopped

Handful arugula

3 sprigs of parsley, chopped

1 tsp extra virgin olive oil

Salt and black pepper

Directions:

Beat the eggs in a small bowl and set aside.

Sauté the shallot for 5 minutes with a bit of the oil, on low-medium heat.

Pour the eggs in the pans, stirring the mixture for just a second.

The eggs on medium heat, and tip the pan just enough to let the loose egg run underneath after about one minute on the burner.

Add the greens, herbs, and the seasonings to the top side as it is still soft.

Tip: you do not even have to flip it, as you can just cook the egg slowly egg as is well (being careful as to not burn).

Tip: Another option is to put it into an oven to broil for 3-5 minutes (checking to make sure it is only until it is golden but burned).

Berry oat breakfast cobbler

Preparation time: 10 minutes | Cooking time: 40 minutes | Servings: 2

Ingredients:

2 cups of oats/flakes that are ready without cooking

1 cup of blackcurrants without the stems

1 tsp of honey (or ¼ tsp of raw sugar)

½ cup of water (add more or less by testing the pan)

1 cup of plain yoghurt (or soy or coconut)

Directions:

Boil the berries, honey and water and then turn it down on low.

Put in a glass container in a refrigerator until it is cool and set (about 30 minutes or more)

When ready to eat, scoop the berries on top of the oats and yoghurt.

Serve immediately.

Pancakes with apples and blackcurrants

Preparation time: 10 minutes | Cooking time: 20 minutes | Servings: 2

Ingredients:

2 apples, cut into small chunks

2 cups of quick cooking oats

1 cup flour of your choice

1 tsp baking powder

2 tbsp raw sugar, coconut sugar, or 2 tbsp honey that is warm and easy to distribute

2 egg whites

1 ¼ cups of milk (or soy/rice/coconut)

2 tsp extra virgin olive oil

A dash of salt

For the berry topping:

1 cup blackcurrants, washed and stalks removed

3 tbsp Water (may use less)

2 tbsp Sugar (see above for types)

Directions:

Place the ingredients for the topping in a small pot simmer, stirring frequently for about 10 minutes until it cooks down and the juices are released.

Take the dry ingredients and mix in a bowl.

After, add the apples and the milk a bit at a time (you may not use it all), until it is a batter.

Stiffly whisk the egg whites and then gently mix them into the pancake batter.

Set aside in the refrigerator.

Pour a one quarter of the oil onto a flat pan or flat griddle, and when hot, pour some of the batter into it in a pancake shape.

When the pancakes start to have golden brown edges and form air bubbles, they may be ready to be gently flipped.

Test to be sure the bottom can life away from the pan before actually flipping.

Repeat for the next three pancakes.

Top each pancake with the berries.

Berry quinoa and chia seed breakfast

Preparation time: 5 minutes | Cooking time: 30 minutes| Servings: 3

Ingredients:

½ cup quinoa

1½ cups milk

2 tbsp chia seeds

¼ cup fresh blueberries or raspberries

2 tbsp pistachios, silvered

Directions:

Combine quinoa and chia seeds with milk and bring to a boil.

Cover, reduce heat and simmer for 15 minutes.

When ready, serve into bowls and top with fresh berries and pistachios.

Sirtfood truffle bites

Preparation time: 10 minutes | Cooking time: 20 minutes |Servings: 2

Ingredients:

1 cup walnuts

¾ cup of Medjool dates, pitted

½ cup of dark chocolate broken into pieces; or cocoa nibs

2 heaping tbsp of cacao powder

½ cup of dried coconut

1 tbsp ground turmeric

1 tbsp extra virgin olive oil, or coconut oil (preferred)

1 tsp vanilla extract, or a vanilla pod, scraped

1 dash of cayenne pepper

1 dash sea salt (up to 1/8 tsp)

2 tbsp water if needed

Directions:

Pulse in a food processor the walnuts and chocolate until finely pulverized.

Gently blend solid ingredients next and the vanilla.

Make a dough.

Make rolled balls out of the dough.

Add water a few drops at a time only if it is necessary.

Do not use too much water, or you will have to go and add more of the other ingredients to compensate.

Refrigerate.

Store for up to a week.

Take them with you to work or when travelling for a quick pick-me-up as well as to quell a sweet tooth.

Spicy kale chips

Preparation time: 10 minutes | Cooking time: 30 minutes | Servings: 2

Ingredients:

1 large head of curly kale, wash, dry and pulled from stem

1 tbsp extra virgin olive oil

Minced parsley

Squeeze of lemon juice

Cayenne pepper (just a pinch)

Dash of soy sauce

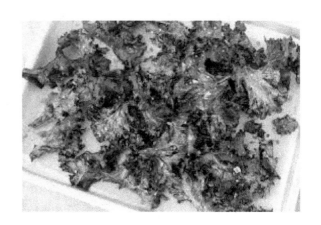

Directions:

In a large bowl, rip the kale from the stem into palm sized pieces.

Sprinkle the minced parsley, olive oil, soy sauce, a squeeze of the lemon juice and a very small pinch of the cayenne powder.

Toss with a set if tongs or salad forks, and make sure to coat all of the leaves.

If you have a dehydrator, turn it on to 118F, spread out the kale on a dehydrator sheet, and leave in there for about 2 hours.

If you are cooking them, place parchment paper on top of a cookie sheet.

Lay the bed of kale and separate it a bit to make sure the kale is evenly toasted.

Cook for 10-15 minutes maximum at 250F.

Sweet and savory guacamole

Preparation time: 10 minutes | Cooking time: 20 minutes | Servings: 2

Ingredients:

2 large avocados, pitted and scooped

2 Medjool dates, pitted and chopped into small pieces

½ cup cherry tomatoes, cut into halves

5 sprigs of parsley, chopped

¼ cup of arugula, chopped

5 sticks of celery, washed, cut into sticks for dipping

Juice from ¼ lime

Dash of sea salt

Directions:

Mash the avocado in a bowl, sprinkle salt, and squeeze of the lime juice.

Fold in the tomatoes, dates, herbs and greens.

Scoop with celery sticks, and enjoy!

Thai nut mix

Preparation time: 10 minutes | Cooking time: 20 minutes | Servings: 2

Ingredients:

½ cup walnuts

½ cup coconut flakes

½ tsp soy sauce

1 tsp honey

1 pinch of cayenne pepper

1 dash of lime juice

Directions:

Add the above ingredients to a bowl, toss the nuts to coat, and place on a baking sheet, lined with parchment paper.

Cook at 250F for 15-20 minutes, checking as not to burn, but lightly toasted.

Remove from oven.

Cool first before eating.

Berry yoghurt freeze

Preparation time: 10 minutes | Cooking time: 25 minutes | Servings: 2

Ingredients:

2 cups plain yoghurt (Greek, soy or coconut)

½ cup sliced strawberries

½ cup blackberries

1 tsp honey (warmed)

½ tsp chocolate powder

Directions:

Blend all of the above ingredients until creamy in a bowl.

Place into two glass or in metal bowls that are freezer-safe, and put into the freezer for 1 hour.

Remove and thaw just slightly so that it is soft enough to eat with a spoon.

Buckwheat pita bread

Preparation time: 10 minutes | Cooking time: 20 minutes | Servings: 2

Ingredients:

1 x 8g packet dried yeast

Polenta for dusting

3 tbsp of olive oil

375ml lukewarm water

500g buckwheat flour

1 tsp of sea salt

Directions:

Combine the yeast and water and let the mixture activate (approximately 10 to 15 minutes).

Combine the buckwheat flour, olive oil, salt and add in the yeast mixture.

Knead it slowly until you make dough.

Cover and place in a warm spot for about an hour (to rise).

Evenly divide the dough into six pieces.

Take a piece, shape it to a flat disc, and then place it in between 2 sheets of baking paper.

Carefully roll out the dough into a ¼-inch thick round pita shapes.

Using a fork, pierce the dough a couple of times and lightly dust it with the polenta.

Heat a 10-inch cast iron and smear it with olive oil.

Cook the bread on one side until puffy then do the same with the other side.

Fill up with desired vegetables and meat and serve immediately.

Alternatively, you could wrap it in foil, place in the fridge, and reheat in the oven the next day.

Smoked salmon omelette

Preparation time: 10 minutes | Cooking time: 10 minutes | Servings: 2

Ingredients:

10g of chopped rocket

100g smoked salmon, sliced

1 tsp of extra virgin olive oil

½ tsp of capers

2 medium eggs

1 tsp of chopped parsley

Directions:

Crack the eggs into a bowl, and whisk them well.

Add the capers, parsley, rocket, and salmon and heat oil in a non-stick pan until hot but not smoking.

Add the egg mixture into the pan and move it around the pan using a spatula.

Reduce the heat to low and let the omelet cook.

Slide the spatula under the omelette, fold it up in half, and serve.

Pancakes with blackcurrant compote

Preparation time: 10 minutes | Cooking time: 30 minutes | Servings: 2

Ingredients:

2 tsp of light olive oil

125g of plain flour

75g of porridge oats

2 apples (peeled, cored and cut into tiny pieces)

1 tsp of baking powder

2 egg whites

Pinch of salt

300ml semi-skimmed milk

2 tbsp of caster sugar

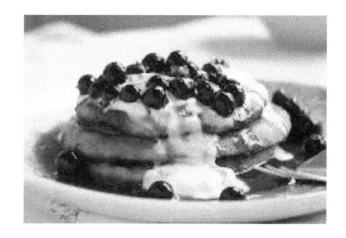

For the compote:

120g blackcurrants, washed and stalks removed

3 tbsp of water

2 tbsp of caster sugar

Directions:

Make the compote first.

Place the blackcurrants, water, and sugar in a small pan.

Bring it to a simmer and let it cook for 10 to 15 minutes.

Place oats, caster sugar, baking powder, flour, and salt in a large bowl and stir well.

Add in the apple then the milk a little at a time as you whisk until you have a smooth batter.

Whisk the egg whites into stiff peaks and fold into the pancake batter.

Transfer the ready batter to a jug.

In a frying pan, placed on medium high heat, heat ½ tsp of oil and add in approximately a quarter of the batter.

Let it cook on both sides until it turns golden brown.

Remove when ready then repeat to make four pancakes.

Drizzle the blackcurrant compote over the pancakes and serve.

Chocolate chips granola

Preparation time: 10 minutes | Cooking time: 30 minutes | Servings: 2

Ingredients:

2 tbsp of rice malt syrup

20g of butter

200g of jumbo oats

60g of good-quality (70%) dark chocolate chips

3 tbsp of light olive oil

1 tbsp of dark brown sugar

50g of roughly chopped pecans

Directions:

Preheat your oven to 160°c.

Use baking parchment or silicone sheet to line a large baking tray.

Add the pecans and oats into a large bowl and mix.

Add butter, olive oil, rice malt syrup, and brown sugar to a small pan and gently heat until the butter melts and the syrup and sugar dissolves (do not allow to boil).

Drizzle the syrup over the oats and stir thoroughly until the oats are fully coated.

Distribute granola all over the baking tray and leave clumps of with a bit of spacing instead of an even spread.

Allow to bake in the oven until you see a tinge of golden brown on the edges (about 20 minutes).

Remove them and allow to cool.

Once cooled, break up the bigger lumps and mix in chocolate chips.

Serve and enjoy.

Scoop the remaining granola into an airtight jar.

It will keep for about 2 weeks.

Breakfast scramble

Preparation time: 10 minutes | Cooking time: 20 minutes | Servings: 2

Ingredients:

A handful of button mushrooms, sliced thinly

1 tsp of mild curry powder

5g of parsley, chopped finely

½ bird's eye chilli, sliced thinly

1 tsp of ground turmeric

2 eggs

1 tsp of extra virgin olive oil

20g kale, chopped roughly

Optional-add seed mixture as toppings and rooster sauce for flavour

Directions:

Mix the curry powder and turmeric, and then add a little water until you have a light paste.

Steam the kale for about 2 to 3 minutes.

Place a frying pan over medium heat and heat the oil.

Fry the mushroom and chilli for 2 to 3 minutes until they start to soften and brown.

Add the paste, cook the eggs, and then serve.

Raspberry and blackcurrant jelly

Preparation time: 10 minutes | Cooking time: 25 minutes | Servings: 2

Ingredients:

100g of raspberries, washed

100g of blackcurrant (washed and stalks removed)

2 leaves of gelatin

300ml water

2 tbsp of granulated sugar

Directions:

Arrange the raspberries in 2 serving glasses or dishes.

Add cold water to a bowl and place the gelatin leaves in so they can soften.

In a small pan, add sugar, 100ml water, and the blackcurrant and boil.

Allow this to simmer for 5 minutes then remove from the heat.

Leave it for 2 minutes then take the gelatin leaves and squeeze out any excess water.

Add the leaves to the saucepan and stir until they fully dissolve.

Add in the rest of the water.

Pour the liquid in prepared dishes and refrigerate.

The jellies will be ready in about 3 to 4 hours overnight.

Strawberry buckwheat tabbouleh

Preparation time: 10 minutes | Cooking time: 20 minutes | Servings: 2

Ingredients:

65g of tomato

1 tbsp of ground turmeric

50g of buckwheat

1 tbsp of extra virgin olive oil

30g of parsley

100g of hulled strawberries

30g of rocket

80g of avocado

20g of red onions

1 tbsp of capers

Juice of ½ lemon

25g of Medjool dates, pitted

Directions:

Cook the buckwheat and the turmeric following the packet directions

Drain, and then set aside to let it cool.

Finely chop the avocado, parsley, red onion, tomato, dates, and capers and mix it with the cool buckwheat.

Slice strawberries and gently mix into the salad together with the lemon juice and oil.

Serve them on a bed of rocket.

Easy quinoa crackers

Preparation time: 10 minutes | Cooking time: 40 minutes | Servings: 2

Ingredients:

2 cups cooked quinoa

1 cup ground flaxseed

2 tbsp sesame seeds

1 tbsp honey

1 tsp salt

1 cup water

3 tbsp extra virgin olive oil

1 tsp garlic powder (optional)

½ tsp dried oregano (optional)

Directions:

Thoroughly mix together all ingredients in a large bowl.

Place the dough on a lined baking sheet and with wet hands, flatten the dough.

Slip the parchment off of the baking sheet, cover the length of the dough with plastic wrap and roll out the dough with a rolling pin to a ¼ inch thickness.

Bake at 350 f for 35 minutes or until the parchment paper easily pulls away and the dough is cooked but not crisp yet.

Flip the cracker over, gently remove the parchment paper and cut into squares.

Bake for another 35 minutes, or until the crackers are nice and crisp.

Granola-the sirt way

Preparation time: 10 minutes | Cooking time: 50 minutes | Servings: 2

Ingredients:

1 cup buckwheat puffs

1 cup buckwheat flakes (ready to eat type, but not whole buckwheat that needs to be cooked)

½ cup coconut flakes

½ cup Medjool dates, without pits, chopped into smaller, bite-sized pieces

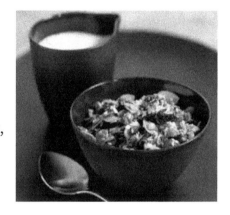

1 cup of cacao nibs or very dark chocolate chips

½ cup walnuts, chopped

1 cup strawberries chopped and without stems

1 cup plain Greek, coconut or soy yoghurt.

Directions:

Mix, without yoghurt and strawberry toppings.

You can store for up to a week. Store in an airtight container.

Add toppings (even different berries or different yoghurt).

You can even use the berry toppings as you will learn how to make from other recipes.

Ginger prawn stir-fry

Preparation time: 10 minutes | Cooking time: 40 minutes | Servings: 2

Ingredients:

6 prawns or shrimp (peeled and deveined)

½ package of buckwheat noodles (called soba in Asian sections)

5-6 leaves of kale, chopped

1 cup of green beans, chopped

5g lovage or celery leaves

1 garlic clove, finely chopped

1 bird's eye chilli, finely chopped

1 tsp fresh ginger, finely chopped

2 stalks celery, chopped

½ small red onion, chopped

1 cup chicken stock (or vegetable if you prefer)

2 tbsp Soy sauce

2 tbsp extra virgin olive oil

Directions:

Cook prawns in a bit of the oil and soy sauce until done and set aside (about 10-15 minutes).

Boil the noodles according the directions (usually 6-8 minutes).

Set aside.

Sauté the vegetables, then add the garlic, ginger, red onion, chilli in a bit of oil until tender and crunchy, but not mushy.

Add the prawns, and noodles, and simmer low about 5-10 minutes past that point.

Chicken with mole salad

Preparation time: 10 minutes | Cooking time: 35 minutes |Servings: 2

Ingredients:

1 skinned chicken breast

2 cups spinach, washed, dried and torn in halves

2 celery stalks, chopped or sliced thinly

½ cup arugula

½ small red onion, diced

2 Medjool pitted dates, chopped

1 tbsp of dark chocolate powder

1 tbsp extra virgin olive oil

2 tbsp Water

5 sprigs of parsley, chopped

Dash of salt

Directions:

In a food processor, blend the dates, chocolate powder, oil and water, and salt.

Add the chilli and process further.

Rub this paste onto the chicken breast, and set it aside, in the refrigerator.

Prepare other salad mixings, the vegetables and herbs in a bowl and toss.

Cook the chicken in a dash of oil in a pan, until done, about 10-15 minutes over a medium burner.

When done, let cool and lay over the salad bed and serve.

Strawberry fields salad

Preparation time: 10 minutes | Cooking time: 20 minutes | Servings: 2

Ingredients:

½ cup cooked buckwheat

1 avocado, pitted, sliced and scooped

1 small tomato, quartered

2 Medjool dates, pitted

5 walnuts, chopped coarsely

20 g red onion

1 tbsp Capers

1 cup arugula

1 cup spinach

3 sprigs parsley, chopped

6 strawberries, sliced

1 tbsp extra virgin olive oil

½ lemon, juiced

1 tbsp Ground turmeric

Directions:

Use room temperature buckwheat or serve warm if preferred.

Wash, dry and chop ingredients above, finish with the lemon and olive oil and turmeric as a dressing.

Add the buckwheat then the strawberries to the top of the salad.

Chilled gazpacho

Preparation time: 10 minutes | Cooking time: 20 minutes | Servings: 2

Ingredients:

2 large, or 6 small tomatoes, chopped

1 avocado, pitted, sliced, and scooped out (wait to do this until instructed)

1 medium cucumber, chopped

1 small red onion, chopped

1 cup of arugula, chopped very finely

½ stalk of celery chopped very finely

1 clove of garlic, minced or pressed

½ chilli or a dash of cayenne pepper

1 tsp lime juice

Dash of sea salt

Dash of pepper

Directions:

Add the ingredients to a blender, or a food processor, and pulse gently.

You do not want to blend too well, or you will make a liquid, as opposed to a soup.

The gazpacho should be chunky.

After blending, put into the refrigerator for about 1 hour.

You can also let this sit overnight.

Just before eating, slice and scoop out the avocado.

Ladle half of the gazpacho into a chilled bowl.

Add the slices of avocado and serve immediately.

Chapter 7: Main dishes

Indian lentil soup

Preparation time: 10 minutes | Cooking time: 50 minutes | Servings: 2

Ingredients:

2 cups of lentils

1 small red onion, minced

1 stalk of celery, finely chopped

1 carrot, chopped

2 large leaves of kale, chopped finely, or 1 cup of baby kale, chopped

2 sprigs of cilantro, minced

3 sprigs of parsley, minced

¼-½ chilli pepper, deseeded and minced (use more or less to your taste)

1 tomato, chopped into small pieces

1 chunk of ginger, minced

1 clove of garlic, minced

5 cups of chicken or vegetable stock

1 tsp of turmeric

1 tsp extra virgin olive oil

½ tsp Salt

Directions:

Cook lentils according to the package, removing from heat about 5 minutes before they would be done.

In a saucepan, sauté all of the vegetables in the olive oil.

Then add the chopped greens last.

Then add the ginger, garlic, and chilli and turmeric powder.

Add the stock and simmer for 5 minutes.

Add the lentils, and salt.

Stir in the precooked lentils and cook longer, on a very low simmer, for 25 more minutes.

Remove from the heat and cool.

Cut the avocado, remove the pit, and slice it, then scoop out the slices just before eating.

Top with avocado slice, then serve immediately.

Shrimp & arugula soup

Preparation time: 5 minutes | Cooking time: 30 minutes | Servings: 3

Ingredients:

10 medium sized shrimp or 5 large prawns, cleaned, deshelled and deveined

1 small red onion, sliced very thinly

1 cup arugula

1 cup baby kale

2 large celery stalks, sliced very thinly

5 sprigs of parsley, chopped

11 cloves of garlic, minced

5 cups of chicken or fish or vegetable stock

1 tbsp extra virgin olive oil

Dash of sea salt

Dash of pepper

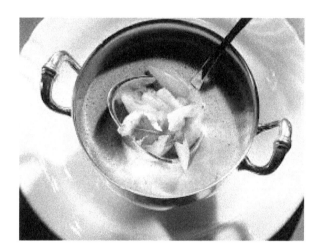

Directions:

Sauté the vegetables (not the kale or arugula just yet however), in a stock pot, on low heat for about 2 minutes so that they are still tender and still crunchy, but not cooked quite yet.

You will need to save the cooking time for the next step.

Add the salt and pepper.

Next, clean and chop the shrimp into bite-sized pieces that would be comfortable eating in a soup.

Then, add the shrimp to the pot, and sauté for 10 more minutes on medium-low heat.

Make sure the shrimp is cooked thoroughly and is not translucent.

When the shrimp seems to be cooked through, add the stock to the pot and cook on medium for about 20 more minutes.

Remove from heat and cool before serving.

Creamy chicken soup

Preparation time: 5 minutes | Cooking time: 30 minutes | Servings: 3

Ingredients:

4 chicken breasts

1 carrot, chopped

1 cup zucchini, peeled and chopped

2 cups cauliflower, broken into florets

1 celery rib, chopped

1 small onion, chopped

5 cups water

½ tsp salt

Black pepper, to taste

Directions:

Place chicken breasts, onion, carrot, celery, cauliflower and zucchini in a deep soup pot.

Add in salt, black pepper and 5 cups of water.

Stir and bring to a boil.

Simmer for 30 minutes then remove chicken from the pot and let it cool slightly.

Blend soup until completely smooth.

Shred or dice the chicken meat, return it back to the pot, stir, and serve.

Broccoli and chicken soup

Preparation time: 5 minutes | Cooking time: 30 minutes | Servings: 3

Ingredients:

4 boneless chicken thighs, diced

1 small carrot, chopped

1 broccoli head, broken into florets

1 garlic clove, chopped

1 small onion, chopped

4 cups water

3 tbsp extra virgin olive oil

½ tsp salt

Black pepper, to taste

Directions:

In a deep soup pot, heat olive oil and gently sauté broccoli for 2-3 minutes, stirring occasionally.

Add in onion, carrot, chicken and cook, stirring, for 2-3 minutes. Stir in salt, black pepper and water.

Bring to a boil. Simmer for 30 minutes then remove from heat and set aside to cool.

In a blender or food processor, blend soup until completely smooth. Serve and enjoy!

Warm chicken and avocado soup

Preparation time: 5 minutes | Cooking time: 30 minutes | Servings: 3

Ingredients:

2 ripe avocados, peeled and chopped

1 cooked chicken breast, shredded

1 garlic clove, chopped

3 cups chicken broth

Salt and black pepper, to taste

Fresh coriander leaves, finely cut, to serve

½ cup sour cream, to serve

Directions:

Combine avocados, garlic, and chicken broth in a blender.

Process until smooth and transfer to a saucepan.

Add in chicken and cook, stirring, over medium heat until the mixture is hot.

Serve topped with sour cream and finely cut coriander leaves.

Healthy chicken and oat soup

Preparation time: 5 minutes | Cooking time: 40 minutes | Servings: 3

Ingredients:

3 chicken breasts, diced

1 small onion, chopped

3 garlic cloves

½ cup quick-cooking oats

1 large carrot, chopped

1 red bell pepper, chopped

1 celery rib, chopped

1 tomato, diced

5 cups water

1 bay leaf

1 tsp salt

½ cup fresh parsley leaves, finely cut

Black pepper, to taste

Directions:

Place the chicken, bay leaf, celery, carrot, onion, red pepper, tomato and salt into a soup pot.

Add in water and bring to the boil then reduce heat and simmer for 30 minutes.

Discard the bay leaf, season with salt and pepper, add in the oats and parsley, simmer for 5 more minutes, and serve.

Asparagus and chicken soup

Preparation time: 5 minutes | Cooking time: 30 minutes | Servings: 3

Ingredients:

2 chicken breast fillets, cooked and diced

2-3 leeks, finely cut

1 bunch asparagus, trimmed and cut

4 cups chicken broth

2 tbsp extra virgin olive oil

½ cup fresh parsley, finely chopped

Salt and black pepper, to taste

Lemon juice, to serve

Directions:

Heat the olive oil in a large soup pot.

Add in the leeks and gently sauté, stirring, for 2-3 minutes.

Add chicken broth, the diced chicken, and bring to a boil.

Reduce heat and simmer for 15 minutes.

Add in asparagus, parsley, salt and black pepper, and cook for 5 minutes more.

Serve with lemon juice.

Mediterranean fish and quinoa soup

Preparation time: 5 minutes | Cooking time: 40 minutes | Servings: 3

Ingredients:

1lb cod fillets, cubed

1 onion, chopped

3 tomatoes, chopped

½ cup quinoa, rinsed

1 red pepper, chopped

1 carrot, chopped

½ cup black olives, pitted and sliced

1 garlic clove, crushed

3 tbsp extra virgin olive oil

A pinch of cayenne pepper

1 bay leaf

1 tsp dried thyme

1 tsp dried dill

½ tsp pepper

½ cup white wine

4 cups water

Salt and black pepper, to taste

½ cup fresh parsley, finely cut

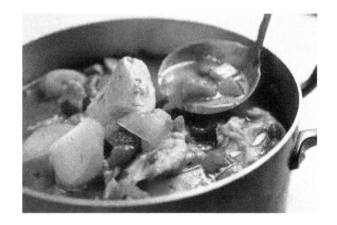

Directions:

Heat the olive oil over medium heat and sauté the onion, red pepper, garlic and carrot until tender.

Stir in the cayenne pepper, bay leaf, herbs, salt and pepper.

Add the white wine, water, quinoa and tomatoes and bring to a boil.

Reduce heat, cover, and cook for 10 minutes.

Stir in olives and the fish and cook for another 10 minutes.

Stir in parsley and serve hot.

Bean stew

Preparation time: 5 minutes | Cooking time: 35 minutes | Servings: 3

Ingredients:

50g of kale, chopped roughly

½ bird's eye chilli, chopped finely (optional)

40g of buckwheat

50g of red onion, chopped finely

1 garlic clove, chopped finely

1 tbsp of roughly chopped parsley

200ml vegetable stock

1 tsp of herbes de provence

200g of tinned mixed beans

1 tsp of tomato purée

1 x 400g tin of chopped Italian tomatoes

30g celery, trimmed and chopped finely

1 tbsp of extra virgin olive oil

30g of carrot, peeled and chopped finely

Directions:

Heat the oil in a medium sized saucepan placed over medium low heat.

Add in the onion, celery, chilli, carrot, garlic and herbs (if using) until the onions are soft enough but not coloured.

Add the stock, tomato purée, and tomatoes and bring to a boil.

Put in the beans and allow for 30 minutes simmering.

Add the kales and cook for 5-10 minutes or until the kale is tender, and then add in parsley.

As it cools, cook the buckwheat as per the directions on the packet.

Drain the buckwheat and serve with the cooked stew.

Pork with pak choi

Preparation time: 5 minutes | Cooking time: 40 minutes | Servings: 3

Ingredients:

100g of shiitake mushrooms, sliced

1 tbsp of corn flour

200g pak choi or choi sum-cut into thin slices

125ml of chicken stock

1 tbsp of tomato purée

1 tsp of brown sugar

1 clove garlic, peeled and crushed

1 shallot, peeled and sliced

100g of bean sprouts

1 tbsp of water

400g of pork mince (10% fat)

1 thumb (5cm) fresh ginger -peeled and grated

400g of firm tofu, cut into large cubes

1 tbsp of rice wine

1 tbsp of soy sauce

A large handful (20g) of parsley, chopped

1 tbsp of rapeseed oil

Directions:

Place the tofu on kitchen paper, cover it with kitchen paper, and then set it aside.

In a small bowl, mix water and corn flour and remove the lumps.

Add in rice wine, brown sugar, chicken stock, tomato puree, and soy sauce.

Also, add in the crushed ginger and garlic them mix.

Place a large frying pan or wok on high heat and add oil to it.

Add the mushrooms and stir-fry for 2 to 3 minutes until cooked and glossy.

Using a slotted spoon, remove the mushrooms from the pan and let them rest.

Add tofu to the pan, fry it until it is brown on all sides, remove it with a slotted spoon when done and set aside.

Add the pak choi to your pan or wok, and stir-fry for about 2 minutes and, then add the mince.

Cook it until it cooks through and then add the sauce.

Reduce the heat a notch and allow the sauce to bubble around the meat for 1-2 minutes.

Add the tofu, beansprouts, and mushrooms to the pan and warm them all through.

Remove it from the heat and mix in parsley then serve right away.

Chicken soup

Preparation time: 5 minutes | Cooking time: 30 minutes | Servings: 3

Ingredients:

1 tsp of smoked paprika	½ tsp of turmeric
300ml passata	30g (large handful) of flat leaf parsley, chopped
Salt and freshly ground black pepper	
1 tsp of dried mixed herbs	1 x 400g can chopped tomatoes
1 x 400g can of black beans, drained	1 tsp of paprika
2 cloves garlic, peeled and crushed	½ tsp of ground cumin
1 carrot, peeled and roughly chopped	1 green pepper, deseeded and chopped
1 litre of water	1 x 400g can kidney beans, drained
1 tsp of mild chilli powder	4 chicken drumsticks
1 red chilli, deseeded then finely chopped	2 shallots, peeled then roughly chopped

Directions:

Take a large saucepan and add in the chicken drumsticks, carrot, and shallots.

Pour in the water and let it simmer.

Allow to cook for 20 minutes, and then remove the chicken drumsticks with a spoon (slotted) and set it aside to cool.

Add in the chopped tomatoes, garlic, passata, chilli, and green pepper, and let it simmer again.

Put in the dried herbs, paprika, turmeric, smoked paprika, chilli powder, and cumin, then simmer again for 30 minutes.

Pull off the skin from the chicken then pinch as much chicken as possible from the bone.

Shred the chicken meat, place it on the pan along with the kidney beans and black beans, and cook for five minutes.

Remove from the heat, add parsley, and stir it in.

Season with pepper and salt (to taste).

Beef with red wine and herb-roasted potatoes

Preparation time: 5 minutes | Cooking time: 60 minutes | Servings: 3

Ingredients:

40ml of red wine

1 tbsp of extra virgin olive oil

1 clove of garlic, finely chopped

5g of parsley, finely chopped

50g of red onions-sliced to rings

50g of sliced kale

1 tsp of corn flour dissolved in 1 tbsp of water

100g of potatoes, peeled then cut into 2cm chunks

150ml of beef stock

1 tsp of tomato purée

150g of beefsteak

Directions:

Preheat your oven to 220 degrees.

Boil the potatoes for 5 minutes then drain.

Place them in a roasting tin together with a tsp of oil and let them roast for 35 to 45 minutes.

Make sure to turn them every ten minutes.

Once done, take them out and mix them with parsley.

Over medium heat, fry the onion in a tsp of oil for 5 to 7 minutes.

Steam the kale for 2 to 3 minutes then drain.

Fry the garlic in a tsp of oil for a minute, add the kale, and stir-fry for 1 to 2 more minutes.

Smear the beef with ½ tsp of oil and fry it in a hot pan over medium heat until cooked as desired.

Remove it and set aside.

Pour wine onto the hot pan and reduce the heat to simmer the wine until syrupy.

Add tomato purée and stock, let it boil, and add the corn flour paste to thicken.

Serve the beef with onion rings, roast potatoes, red wine sauce, kale, and enjoy.

Salmon salad with mint dressing

Preparation time: 5 minutes | Cooking time: 30 minutes | Servings: 3

Ingredients:

1 small handful (10g) of parsley, chopped roughly

2 radishes, trimmed and thinly sliced

40g of young spinach leaves

5cm piece (50g) cucumber, cut into chunks

40g of mixed salad leaves

2 spring onions, trimmed then sliced

1 salmon fillet (130g)

For the dressing:

1 tbsp of rice vinegar

1 tsp of low-fat mayonnaise

Salt and freshly ground black pepper, to taste

2mint leaves, finely chopped

1 tbsp of natural yoghurt

Directions:

Preheat your oven to 200 degrees. Place salmon fillets on a baking tray and allow them to bake for about 16-18 minutes.

Remove from the oven and then let them rest (salmon is ok served hot or cold when added to the salad).

Remove the skin of your salmon (if it has one) after cooking.

Mix the mayonnaise, mint leaves, rice wine vinegar, salt, yoghurt, and pepper in a small bowl and let it stand for 5 minutes to let the flavour deepen.

Place the salad leaves with the spinach on top of a plate and top with the radishes, spring onions, cucumber, and parsley.

Flake the salmon onto the salad then drizzle the dressing over.

Hearty quinoa and spinach breakfast casserole

Preparation time: 5 minutes | Cooking time: 20 minutes | Servings: 3

Ingredients:

1 cup cooked quinoa

3-4 spring onions, finely chopped

5 oz frozen chopped spinach, thawed and squeezed dry

½ zucchini, peeled and shredded

5 eggs

½ cup milk

4 tbsp extra virgin olive oil

salt and black pepper, to taste

1 cup cheddar cheese, grated

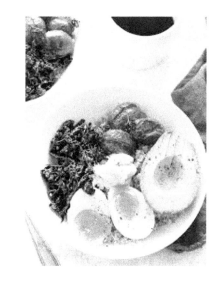

Directions:

In a large bowl combine eggs, milk, salt and pepper.

In a deep casserole dish heat the olive oil.

Cook the onions, zucchini and spinach, stirring constantly, until lightly cooked.

Add in the quinoa and combine everything well.

Pour the egg mixture over and then top with cheddar cheese.

Bake in a preheated to 350 f oven for 20 minutes.

Quick quinoa vegetable scramble

Preparation time: 5 minutes | Cooking time: 30 minutes | Servings: 3

Ingredients:

½ cup cooked quinoa

½ small onion, chopped

2 tomatoes, diced

1 large red pepper, chopped

5 eggs

½ cup crumbled feta

4 tbsp extra virgin olive oil

Black pepper, to taste

Salt, to taste

Directions:

In a large pan, sauté onion over medium heat for 1-2 minutes, stirring.

Add in tomatoes and red pepper and cook until the mixture is almost dry.

Stir in quinoa, feta and eggs and cook until well mixed and not too liquid.

Season with black pepper and serve.

Coconut and quinoa banana pudding

Preparation time: 5 minutes | Cooking time: 30 minutes | Servings: 3

Ingredients:

1 cup quinoa

3 cups coconut milk

3 ripe bananas

¼ cup flaked unsweetened coconut

4 tbsp sugar

1 tsp vanilla extract

Directions:

Wash and cook quinoa according to package directions.

When ready remove from heat and set aside.

In a separate bowl blend sugar, milk and bananas until smooth.

Add to the quinoa.

Heat over medium heat, string, until creamy.

Stir in vanilla and coconut flakes and serve warm.

Chicken with kale and chilli salsa

Preparation time: 5 minutes | Cooking time: 40 minutes| Servings: 3

Ingredients:

50g of buckwheat

1 tsp of chopped fresh ginger

Juice of ½ lemon, divided

2 tsp of ground turmeric

50g of kale, chopped

20g red onion, sliced

120g of skinless, boneless chicken breast

1 tbsp of extra virgin olive oil

1 tomato

1 handful parsley

1 bird's eye chilli, chopped

Directions:

Start with the salsa: remove the eye out of the tomato and finely chop it, making sure to keep as much of the liquid as you can.

Mix it with the chilli, parsley, and lemon juice.

You could add everything to a blender for different results.

Heat your oven to 220F.

Marinate the chicken with a little oil, 1 tsp of turmeric, and the lemon juice.

Let it rest for 5-10 minutes.

Heat a pan over medium heat until it is hot then add marinated chicken and allow it to cook for a minute on both sides until it is pale gold).

Transfer the chicken to the oven (if pan is not ovenproof place it in a baking tray) and bake for 8 to 10 minutes or until it is cooked through.

Take the chicken out of the oven, cover with foil, and let it rest for five minutes before you serve.

Meanwhile, in a steamer, steam the kale for about 5 minutes.

In a little oil, fry the ginger and red onions until they are soft but not coloured, and then add in the cooked kale and fry it for a minute.

Cook the buckwheat in accordance to the packet directions with the remaining turmeric.

Serve alongside the vegetables, salsa and chicken.

Sirt salmon salad

Preparation time: 5 minutes | Cooking time: 30 minutes | Servings: 3

Ingredients:

1 large Medjool date, pitted then chopped

50g of chicory leaves

50g of rocket

1 tbsp of extra virgin olive oil

10g of parsley, chopped

10g of celery leaves, chopped

40g of celery, sliced

15g of walnuts, chopped

1 tbsp of capers

20g of red onions-sliced

80g of avocado-peeled, stoned, and sliced

Juice of ¼ lemon

100g of smoked salmon slices (alternatives: lentils, tinned tuna, or cooked chicken breast)

Directions:

Arrange all the salad leaves on a large plate then mix the rest of the ingredients and distribute evenly on top the leaves.

Greek salad skewers

Preparation time: 5 minutes | Cooking time: 30 minutes | Servings: 3

Ingredients:

100g of cucumber, cut into 4 slices and halved (about 10cm)

8 cherry tomatoes

100g feta, cut into 8 cubes

8 large black olives

1 yellow pepper, cut into 8 squares

½ red onion, cut in half and separated into 8 pieces

2 wooden skewers, soaked in water for 30 minutes before use

For the dressing:

Juice of ½ lemon

½ garlic clove, peeled and crushed

1 tbsp of extra virgin olive oil

A few leaves of finely chopped basil

Generous seasoning of salt and freshly ground black pepper

a few finely chopped oregano leaves

1 tsp of balsamic vinegar

Directions:

Thread every skewer with salad ingredients in this order; olive, followed by tomato, then yellow pepper, red onion, followed by cucumber then feta, tomato, olive, then yellow pepper, red onion and finally cucumber.

Place the dressing ingredients in a small bowl, mix them thoroughly, and then pour over the skewers.

Alkalizing green soup

Preparation time: 5 minutes | Cooking time: 40 minutes | Servings: 3

Ingredients:

2 cups broccoli, cut into florets and chopped

2 zucchinis, peeled and chopped

2 cups chopped kale

1 small onion, chopped

2-3 garlic cloves, chopped

4 cups vegetable broth

2 tbsp extra virgin olive oil

½ tsp ground ginger

½ tsp ground coriander

1 lime, juiced, to serve

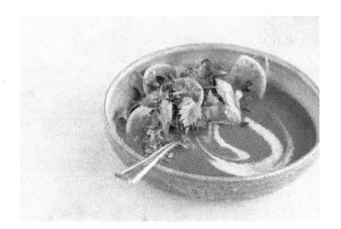

Directions:

Gently heat olive oil in a large saucepan over medium-high heat.

Cook onion and garlic for 3-4 minutes until tender.

Add ginger and coriander and stir to coat well.

Add in broccoli, zucchinis, kale and vegetable broth.

Bring to the boil, then reduce heat and simmer for 15 minutes, stirring from time to time.

Set aside to cool and blend until smooth.

Return to pan and cook until heated through. Serve with lime juice.

Creamy broccoli and potato soup

Preparation time: 5 minutes | Cooking time: 30 minutes | Servings: 3

Ingredients:

3 cups broccoli, cut into florets and chopped

2 potatoes, peeled and chopped

1 large onion, chopped

3 garlic cloves, minced

1 cup raw cashews

1 cup vegetable broth

4 cups water

3 tbsp extra virgin olive oil

½ tsp ground nutmeg

Directions:

Soak cashews in a bowl covered with water for at least 4 hours.

Drain water and blend cashews with 1 cup of vegetable broth until smooth.

Set aside.

Gently heat olive oil in a large saucepan over medium-high heat.

Cook onion and garlic for 3-4 minutes until tender.

Add in broccoli, potato, nutmeg and water.

Cover and bring to the boil, then reduce heat and simmer for 20 minutes, stirring from time to time.

Remove from heat and stir in cashew mixture.

Blend until smooth, return to pan and cook until heated through.

Creamy brussels sprout soup

Preparation time: 5 minutes | Cooking time: 35 minutes | Servings: 3

Ingredients:

1lb frozen brussels sprouts, thawed

2 potatoes, peeled and chopped

1 large onion, chopped

3 garlic cloves, minced

1 cup raw cashews

4 cups vegetable broth

3 tbsp extra virgin olive oil

½ tsp curry powder

Salt and black pepper, to taste

Directions:

Soak cashews in a bowl covered with water for at least 4 hours.

Drain water and blend cashews with 1 cup of vegetable broth until smooth.

Set aside.

Gently heat olive oil in a large saucepan over medium-high heat.

Cook onion and garlic and for 3-4 minutes until tender.

Add in brussels sprouts, potato, curry and vegetable broth.

Cover and bring to a boil, then reduce heat and simmer for 20 minutes, stirring from time to time.

Remove from heat and stir in cashew mixture.

Blend until smooth, return to pan and cook until heated through.

Chicken and arugula salad with Italian dressing

Preparation time: 5 minutes | Cooking time: 30 minutes | Servings: 3

Ingredients:

6oz. of chicken (or turkey), skinless, boneless grilled or prepared in the skillet

Large mixed arugula and lettuce salad

½ cup Italian dressing

½ tsp of mustard

Tuna with arugula salad with Italian dressing

6 oz. Can of tuna, drained.

Large mixed arugula

Red onion salad

½ cup italian dressing

½ tsp of mustard

You may use fish sauce instead of salt

Avocado and chicken risotto

Preparation time: 5 minutes | Cooking time: 20 minutes | Servings: 3

Ingredients:

3 cups chicken broth

2 chicken breasts, diced

1 cup risotto rice

2 avocados, peeled and diced

3 tbsp extra virgin olive oil

1 onion, finely chopped

2 garlic cloves, crushed

2 tbsp raisins

1 cup grated parmesan cheese, plus extra to serve

5-6 green onions, finely cut, to serve

Directions:

Place chicken broth in a saucepan, bring to the boil, then reduce heat to low and keep at a simmer.

In a non-stick fry pan, cook chicken for 5-6 minutes each side, or until browned and cooked through.

Transfer to a plate in the same pan, heat olive oil over medium heat.

Add the onion and cook, stirring, for 1-2 minutes until softened.

Stir in the garlic, then add the rice and cook, stirring, for 1 minute to coat the grains.

Add the broth, a spoonful at a time, stirring occasionally, allowing each spoonful to be absorbed before adding the next.

Simmer until all liquid has absorbed and rice is tender.

Stir in the chicken, parmesan cheese and raisins, then cover and remove from the heat.

Serve in bowls topped with diced avocados, extra parmesan cheese and chopped green onions.

Chicken and chickpea fritters

Preparation time: 5 minutes | Cooking time: 30 minutes | Servings: 3

Ingredients:

1 can chickpeas, drained

2 chicken breasts, cooked and shredded

2 egg whites

½ cup fresh parsley leaves, very finely cut

1 tsp ginger

½ tsp black pepper salt, to taste

2 tbsp coconut oil, for frying

Directions:

Blend the chickpeas in a food processor and combine them with the chicken, egg whites, parsley, and ginger into a smooth batter.

Heat the oil in a frying pan over medium heat.

Using a large tbsp, form the batter into fritters.

Cook each one for 2-3 minutes each side or until golden and cooked through.

Chicken and lentil stew

Preparation time: 5 minutes | Cooking time: 50 minutes | Servings: 3

Ingredients:

4 chicken breasts, diced

½ cup red lentils, rinsed

1 carrot, chopped

1 small onion, chopped

1 garlic clove, chopped

1 celery stalk, chopped

1 small red pepper, chopped

1 can tomatoes, chopped

1 tbsp paprika

1 tsp ginger, grated

3 tbsp extra virgin olive oil

½ cup fresh parsley leaves, finely cut, to serve

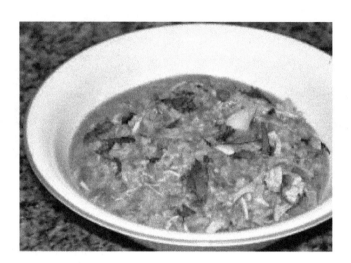

Directions:

Heat olive oil in a casserole and gently brown the chicken, stirring.

Add in onions, garlic, celery, carrot, pepper, paprika and ginger.

Cook, stirring constantly, for 2-3 minutes.

Add in the lentils and tomatoes and bring to a boil.

Lower heat, cover, and simmer for 30 minutes, or until the lentils are tender and the chicken is cooked through.

Serve sprinkled with fresh parsley.

Brussels sprouts egg skillet

Preparation time: 5 minutes | Cooking time: 30 minutes | Servings: 3

Ingredients:

½lb brussels sprouts, halved

1 small onion, chopped

10 cherry tomatoes, halved

4 eggs

1 tbsp extra virgin olive oil

Directions:

In an 8 inch cast iron skillet, heat olive oil over medium heat.

Add in onion and sauté for 1-2 minutes.

Add in brussels sprouts and tomatoes and season with salt and pepper to taste.

Cook for 3-4 minutes then crack the eggs, cover and cook until egg whites have set, and egg yolk is desired consistency.

Salmon kebabs

Preparation time: 5 minutes | Cooking time: 20 minutes | Servings: 3

Ingredients:

2 shallots, ends trimmed, halved

2 zucchinis, cut in 2-inch cubes

1 cup cherry tomatoes

6 skinless salmon fillets, cut into 1-inch pieces

3 limes, cut into thin wedges

Directions:

Preheat barbecue or char grill on medium-high.

Thread fish cubes onto skewers, then zucchinis, shallots and tomatoes.

Repeat to make 12 kebabs.

Bake the kebabs for about 3 minutes each side for medium cooked.

Transfer to a plate, cover with foil and set aside for 5 min to rest.

Mediterranean baked salmon

Preparation time: 5 minutes | Cooking time: 30 minutes | Servings: 3

Ingredients:

2 (6 oz) boneless salmon fillets

1 tomato, thinly sliced

1 onion, thinly sliced

1 tbsp capers

3 tbsp olive oil

1 tsp dry oregano

3 tbsp parmesan cheese

Salt and black pepper, to taste

Directions:

Preheat oven to 350F.

Place the salmon fillets in a baking dish, sprinkle with oregano, top with onion and tomato slices, drizzle with olive oil, and sprinkle with capers and parmesan cheese.

Cover the dish with foil and bake for 30 minutes, or until the fish flakes easily.

Simple oven-baked sea bass

Preparation time: 5 minutes | Cooking time: 50 minutes | Servings: 3

Ingredients:

1lb sea bass, cleaned and scaled

5 oz fennel, trimmed and sliced

5-6 spring onions, chopped

2 garlic cloves, chopped

10 black olives, pitted and halved

2-3 lemon wedges

1 tbsp capers

2 garlic cloves, finely chopped

½ tsp paprika

½ cup dry white wine

3 tbsp extra virgin olive oil

Salt and pepper, to taste

Directions:

In a cup, mix garlic, olive oil, salt, and black pepper.

Arrange the sliced fennel in a shallow ovenproof casserole.

Add the green onions and lay the fish on top.

Pour over the olive mixture.

Scatter the olives, paprika and lemon wedges over the fish, then pour the wine over.

Cover the dish with a lid or foil and bake for 20 minutes, or until the fish flakes easily.

Lemon rosemary fish fillets

Preparation time: 5 minutes | Cooking time: 30 minutes | Servings: 3

Ingredients:

4 white fish fillets

1 tbsp dried rosemary

4 tbsp breadcrumbs

2 tbsp lemon zest

1 tsp garlic powder

2 tbsp extra virgin olive oil

1 tsp salt

Directions:

Combine the rosemary, breadcrumbs, lemon zest, garlic powder and salt in a food processor and blend until well mixed.

Place the fish fillets, skin-side up, on a lined baking tray.

Grill for 3-4 minutes.

Turn the fish over and press a quarter of the breadcrumb mixture over the top of each fillet.

Drizzle with olive oil and grill for 4 min until the crust is golden and the fish is cooked through.

Serve with steamed spinach or baked potatoes.

Asian salmon with broccoli

Preparation time: 5 minutes | Cooking time: 40 minutes | Servings: 3

Ingredients:

4 salmon fillets, skin on

1 lb fresh broccoli florets

2 tbsp soy sauce

2 tbsp toasted sesame oil

1 tsp chilli garlic sauce

1 tbsp brown sugar

½ cup green onions, finely cut, to serve

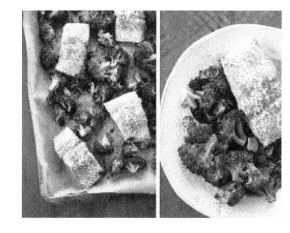

Directions:

In a large bowl, combine the garlic and soy sauce with the sesame oil and brown sugar.

Add in the salmon and broccoli and toss to coat.

Place salmon skin side down in a single layer on a lined baking tray.

Add the broccoli florets around.

Bake 10-12 minutes or until the fish is cooked through and flakes easily with a fork.

Top with green onions and serve.

Salmon and spinach with feta cheese

Preparation time: 5 minutes | Cooking time: 30 minutes | Servings: 3

Ingredients:

4 salmon fillets, skin on

1 bag frozen spinach

4-5 green onions, chopped

1 cup crumbled feta cheese

4 tbsp extra virgin olive oil

Salt and pepper, to taste

Lemon wedges, to serve

Directions:

In a skillet, heat olive oil on medium-high.

Cook the spinach and the green onions for 2-3 min, stirring once or twice.

Season with salt and pepper to taste and add in the feta cheese.

Cook for 1 minute more.

Place salmon skin side down in a single layer on a lined baking tray and roast for 10-12 minutes or until it is cooked through and flakes easily with a fork.

Spoon the spinach mixture onto plates, then top with the salmon and serve with lemon wedges.

Chapter 8: Snacks and juices

Sirt fruit salad

Preparation time: 5 minutes | Cooking time: 0 minutes |Servings: 3

Ingredients:

½ cup crisply made green tea

1 tsp nectar

1 orange, divided

1 apple, cored and generally slashed

10 red seedless grapes

10 blueberries

Directions:

Stir the nectar into a large portion of some green tea.

When broken down, include the juice of a large portion of the orange.

Leave to cool.

Chop the other portion of the orange and spot in a bowl together with the cleaved apple, grapes and blueberries.

Pour over the cooled tea and leave to soak for a couple of moments before serving.

Raspberry and blackcurrant jelly

Preparation time: 5 minutes | Cooking time: 0 minutes | Servings: 3

Ingredients:

100g raspberries, washed

2 leaves gelatine

100g blackcurrants, washed and stalks evacuated

2 tbsp granulated sugar

300ml water

Directions:

Arrange the raspberries in two serving dishes/glasses/moulds.

Put the gelatine leaves in a bowl of cold water to soften.

Place the blackcurrants in a little container with the sugar and 100ml water and bring to the bubble.

Stew vivaciously for 5 minutes and afterward expel from the warmth.

Leave to represent 2 minutes.

Squeeze out overabundance water from the gelatine leaves and add them to the pot.

Mix until completely broke up, then mix in the remainder of the water.

Empty the fluid into the readied dishes and refrigerate to set.

The jams ought to be prepared in around 3-4 hours or medium-term.

Apple pancakes with blackcurrant compote

Preparation time: 5 minutes | Cooking time: 20 minutes | Servings: 3

Ingredients:

75g porridge oats sirtfood plans

125g plain flour

1 tsp heating powder

2 tbsp caster sugar

Spot of salt

2 apples, stripped, cored and cut into little pieces

300ml semi-skimmed milk

2 egg whites

2 tsp light olive oil

For the compote:

120g blackcurrants, washed and stalks expelled

2 tbsp caster sugar

3 tbsp water

Directions:

First make the compote.

Spot the blackcurrants, sugar and water in a little dish.

Raise to a stew and cook for 10-15 minutes.

Place the oats, flour, heating powder, caster sugar and salt in a huge bowl and blend well.

Mix in the apple and afterward rush in the milk a little at once until you have a smooth blend.

Whisk the egg whites to stiff pinnacles and afterward crease into the hotcake player.

Move the player to a container.

Heat ½ tsp oil in a non-stick skillet on a medium-high warmth and pour in around one fourth of the hitter.

Cook on the two sides until brilliant dark coloured. Evacuate and rehash to make four hotcakes.

Serve the flapjacks with the blackcurrant compote sprinkled over

Quinoa and date cookies

Preparation time: 5 minutes | Cooking time: 30 minutes | Servings: 3

Ingredients:

½ cup almond flour

½ cup cooked quinoa

1/3 cup brown sugar

½ cup butter

4 tbsp tahini

16 dates, pitted and chopped

1 tsp baking soda

½ tsp vanilla extract

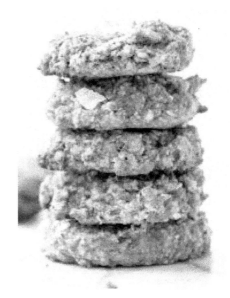

Directions:

Preheat oven to 350F.

Combine sugar, tahini and butter stirring until creamy.

Add in remaining

Ingredients. Mix very well.

Spoon rounded teaspoonfuls of dough onto cookie sheets.

Bake for 10-12 minutes, or until cookies start to turn golden brown.

The sirtfood diet green juice

Preparation time: 5 minutes | Cooking time: 0 minutes | Servings: 3

Ingredients:

(2 enormous bunches) kale

30 g (an enormous bunch) rocket

5 g (a little bunch) level leaf parsley

5 g (a little bunch) lovage leaves (discretionary)

Enormous stalks green celery, including leaves

A large portion of a medium green apple

A large portion of a lemon, squeezed

Matcha green tea

Directions:

Blend the greens (kale, rocket, parsley, and lovage, on the off chance that utilizing) together, at that point juice them.

We discover juicers can truly vary in their proficiency at squeezing verdant vegetables and you may need to re-squeeze the leftovers before proceeding onward to different fixings.

The objective is to wind up with about 50ml of juice from the greens.

Presently squeeze the celery and the apple

You can strip the lemon and put it through the juicer also, however, we think that it's a lot simpler to just press the lemon by hand into the juice.

By this stage, you ought to have around 250ml of juice altogether, maybe somewhat more.

It is just when the juice is made and prepared to serve that you include the matcha green tea.

Pour a modest quantity of the juice into a glass, at that point include the matcha and mix vivaciously with a fork or tsp.

We just use matcha in the initial two beverages of the day as it contains moderate measures of caffeine (a similar substance as a typical cup of tea).

For individuals not accustomed to it, it might keep them alert whenever alcoholic late.

Once the match is broken down include the rest of the juice.

Give it a last mix, at that point, your juice is prepared to drink.

Don't hesitate to top up with plain water, as indicated by taste.

Kale and blackcurrant smoothie

Preparation time: 5 minutes | Cooking time: 0 minutes | Servings: 3

Ingredients:

2 tsp nectar

1 cup crisply made green tea

10 infant kale leaves, stalks evacuated

1 ready banana

40 g blackcurrants, washed and stalks evacuated

6 ice solid shapes

Directions:

Mix the nectar into the warm green tea until broke down.

Wonder every one of the fixings together in a blender until smooth.

Serve right away.

Green tea smoothie

Preparation time: 5 minutes | Cooking time: 0 minutes | Servings: 3

Ingredients:

2 ready bananas

250 ml milk

2 tsp matcha green tea powder

½ tsp vanilla bean glue (not separate) or a little scratch of the seeds from a vanilla unit

6 ice 3D squares

2 tsp nectar

Directions:

Mix every one of the fixings together in a blender and serve in two glasses.

Raw vegan fruits dipped in superfoods chocolate

Preparation time: 5 minutes | Cooking time: 0 minutes | Servings: 3

Ingredients:

2 apples or 2 bananas or a bowl of strawberries or any fruit that can be dipped in melted chocolate

½ cup of melted superfoods chocolate (see earlier recipe)

2 tbsp chopped nuts (almond, walnut, brazil nuts) or seeds (hemp, chia, sesame, flax meal)

Directions:

Cut apple in wedges or cut banana in quarters.

Melt the chocolate and chop the nuts.

Dip fruit in chocolate, sprinkle with nuts or seeds and lay on tray.

Transfer the tray to the fridge so the chocolate can harden; serve.

If you don't want chocolate, cover fruits with almond or sunflower butter and sprinkle with chia or hemp seeds, cut it into chunks and serve.

Fruit skewers & strawberry dip

Preparation time: 5 minutes| Cooking time: 0 minutes| Servings: 3

Ingredients:

150g (5oz) red grapes

1 pineapple, (approx. 2lb weight) peeled and diced

400g (14oz) strawberries

Directions:

Place 100g (3½ oz) of the strawberries into a food processor and blend until smooth.

Pour the dip into a serving bowl.

Skewer the grapes, pineapple chunks and remaining strawberries onto skewers.

Serve alongside the strawberry dip.

Choc nut truffles

Preparation time: 5 minutes | Cooking time: 0 minutes | Servings: 3

Ingredients:

150g (5oz) desiccated (shredded) coconut

50g (2oz) walnuts, chopped

25g (1oz) hazelnuts, chopped

4 Medjool dates

2 tbsp 100% cocoa powder or cacao nibs

1 tbsp coconut oil

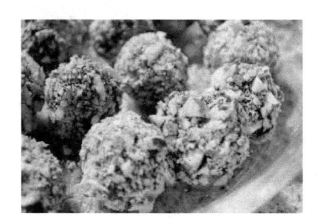

Directions:

Place all of the ingredients into a blender and process until smooth and creamy.

Using a tsp, scoop the mixture into bite-size pieces then roll it into balls.

Place them into small paper cases, cover them and chill for 1 hour before serving.

No-bake strawberry flapjacks

Preparation time: 5 minutes | Cooking time: 30 minutes | Servings: 3

Ingredients:

75g (3oz) porridge oats

125g (4oz) dates

50g (2oz) strawberries

50g (2oz) peanuts (unsalted)

50g (2oz) walnuts

1 tbsp coconut oil

2 tbsp 100% cocoa powder or cacao nibs

Directions:

Place all of the ingredients into a blender and process until they become a soft consistency.

Spread the mixture onto a baking sheet or small flat tin.

Press the mixture down and smooth it out.

Cut it into 8 pieces, ready to serve.

You can add an extra sprinkling of cocoa powder to garnish if you wish.

Chocolate balls

Preparation time: 5 minutes | Cooking time: 10 minutes | Servings: 3

Ingredients:

50g (2oz) peanut butter (or almond butter)

25g (1oz) cocoa powder

25g (1oz) desiccated (shredded) coconut

1 tbsp honey

1 tbsp cocoa powder for coating

Directions:

Place the ingredients into a bowl and mix.

Using a tsp scoop out a little of the mixture and shape it into a ball.

Roll the ball in a little cocoa powder and set aside.

Repeat for the remaining mixture.

Can be eaten straight away or stored in the fridge.

Warm berries & cream

Preparation time: 5 minutes | Cooking time: 0 minutes | Servings: 3

Ingredients

250g (9oz) blueberries

250g (9oz) strawberries

100g (3½ oz) redcurrants

100g (3½ oz) blackberries

4 tbsp fresh whipped cream

1 tbsp honey

Zest and juice of 1 orange

Directions

Place all of the berries into a pan along with the honey and orange juice.

Gently heat the berries for around 5 minutes until warmed through.

Serve the berries into bowls and add a dollop of whipped cream on top.

Alternatively, you could top them off with fromage frais or yoghurt.

Chocolate fondue

Preparation time: 5 minutes | Cooking time: 10 minutes | Servings: 3

Ingredients:

125g (4oz) dark chocolate (min 85% cocoa)

300g (11oz) strawberries

200g (7oz) cherries

2 apples, peeled, cored and sliced

100ml (3½ fl oz) double cream (heavy cream)

Directions:

Place the chocolate and cream into a fondue pot or saucepan and warm it until smooth and creamy.

Serve in the fondue pot or transfer it to a serving bowl.

Scatter the fruit on a serving dish ready to be dipped into the chocolate.

Walnut & date loaf

Preparation time: 5 minutes | Cooking time: 30 minutes | Servings: 3

Ingredients:

250g (9oz) self-rising flour

125g (4oz) Medjool dates, chopped

50g (2oz) walnuts, chopped

250ml (8fl oz) milk

3 eggs

1 medium banana, mashed

1 tsp baking soda

Directions:

Sieve the baking soda and flour into a bowl.

Add in the banana, eggs, milk and dates and combine all the ingredients thoroughly.

Transfer the mixture to a lined loaf tin and smooth it out.

Scatter the walnuts on top.

Bake the loaf in the oven at 180C/360F for 45 minutes.

Transfer it to a wire rack to cool before serving.

Strawberry frozen yoghurt

Preparation time: 5 minutes | Cooking time: 0 minutes | Servings: 3

Ingredients:

450g (1lb) plain yoghurt

175g (6oz) strawberries juice of

1 orange

1 tbsp honey

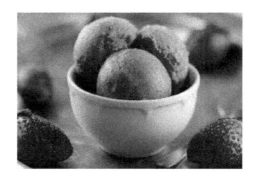

Directions:

Place the strawberries and orange juice into a food processor or blender and blitz until smooth.

Press the mixture through a sieve into a large bowl to remove seeds.

Stir in the honey and yoghurt.

Transfer the mixture to an ice-cream maker and follow the manufacturer's directions.

Alternatively pour the mixture into a container and place in the fridge for 1 hour.

Use a fork to whisk it and break up ice crystals and freeze for 2 hours.

Chocolate brownies

Preparation time: 5 minutes | Cooking time: 30 minutes | Servings: 3

Ingredients:

200g (7oz) dark chocolate (min 85% cocoa)

200g (7oz) Medjool dates, stone removed

100g (3½oz) walnuts, chopped

3 eggs

25ml (1fl oz) melted coconut oil

2 tsp vanilla essence

½ tsp baking soda

Makes 14 197 calories per serving

Directions:

Place the dates, chocolate, eggs, coconut oil, baking soda and vanilla essence into a food processor and mix until smooth.

Stir the walnuts into the mixture.

Pour the mixture into a shallow baking tray.

Transfer to the oven and bake at 180C/350F for 25-30 minutes.

Allow it to cool.

Cut into pieces and serve.

Crème brûlée

Preparation time: 5 minutes | Cooking time: 0 minutes | Servings: 3

Ingredients:

400g (14oz) strawberries

300g (11oz) plain low-fat yoghurt

125g (4oz) Greek yoghurt

100g (3½oz) brown sugar

1 tsp vanilla extract

Directions:

Divide the strawberries between 4 ramekin dishes.

In a bowl combine the plain yoghurt with the vanilla extract.

Spoon the mixture onto the strawberries. Scoop the Greek yoghurt on top.

Sprinkle the sugar into each ramekin dish, completely covering the top.

Place the dishes under a hot grill (broiler) for around 3 minutes or until the sugar has caramelised.

Pistachio fudge

Preparation time: 5 minutes | Cooking time: 0 minutes| Servings: 3

Ingredients:

225g (8oz) Medjool dates

100g (3½ oz) pistachio nuts, shelled

(or other nuts)

50g (2oz) desiccated (shredded) coconut

25g (1oz) oats

2 tbsp water

Directions:

Place the dates, nuts, coconut, oats and water into a food processor and process until the ingredients are well mixed.

Remove the mixture and roll it to 2cm (1 inch) thick.

Cut it into 10 pieces and serve.

Spiced poached apples

Preparation time: 5 minutes | Cooking time: 0 minutes | Servings: 3

Ingredients:

4 apples

2 tbsp honey

4 star-anises

2 cinnamon sticks

300ml (½ pint) green tea

Directions:

Place the honey and green tea into a saucepan and bring to the boil.

Add the apples, star anise and cinnamon.

Reduce the heat and simmer gently for 15 minutes.

Serve the apples with a dollop of crème fraiche or Greek yoghurt.

Black forest smoothie

Preparation time: 5 minutes | Cooking time: 0 minutes | Servings: 3

Ingredients

100g (3½oz) frozen cherries

25g (1oz) kale

1 Medjool date

1 tbsp cocoa powder

2 tsp chia seeds

200ml (7fl oz) milk or soya milk

Directions

Place all the ingredients into a blender and process until smooth and creamy.

Creamy coffee smoothie

Preparation time: 5 minutes | Cooking time: 0 minutes| Servings: 3

Ingredients:

1 banana

1 tsp chia seeds

1 tsp coffee

½ avocado

120ml (4fl oz) water

Serves 1

239 calories per serving

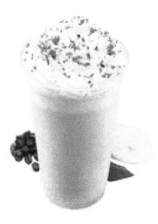

Directions:

Place all the ingredients into a food processor or blender and blitz until smooth.

You can add a little crushed ice too.

This can also double as a breakfast smoothie.

Grape and melon smoothie

Preparation time: 5 minutes | Cooking time: 0 minutes | Servings: 3

Ingredients:

100g of cantaloupe melon

100g of red seedless grapes

30g of young spinach leaves, stalks removed

½ cucumber

Directions:

Peel the cucumber, then cut it into half.

Remove the seeds and chop it roughly.

Peel the cantaloupe, deseed it, and cut it into chunks.

Place all ingredients in a blender and blend until smooth.

Sirt energy balls

Preparation time: 5 minutes | Cooking time: 40 minutes | Servings: 3

Ingredients:

1 mug of mixed nuts (with plenty of walnuts)

7 Medjool dates

1 tbsp of coconut oil

2 tbsp of cocoa powder

zest of 1 orange (optional)

Directions:

Start by placing the nuts in a food processor and grind them until almost powdered (more or less depending on the preferred texture of your energy balls).

Add the Medjool dates, coconut oil, cacao powder, and run the blender again until fully mixed.

Place the blend in a refrigerator for half an hour, and then shape them into balls.

You can add in the zest of an orange as you blend.

Cupcakes with matcha icing

Preparation time: 5 minutes | Cooking time: 50 minutes | Servings: 3

Ingredients:

½ tsp of salt

200g of caster sugar

½ tsp of vanilla extract

150g of self-rising flour

60g of cocoa

1 egg

120ml milk

½ tsp of fine espresso coffee, decaf if preferred

120ml of boiling water

50ml of vegetable oil

For the icing:

1 tbsp of matcha green tea powder

50g of at room temperature butter

50g of icing sugar

½ tsp of vanilla bean paste

50g of soft cream cheese

Directions:

Heat the oven to 160-180C fan.

Line a cupcake tin with silicone cake cases or paper.

Thoroughly mix salt, flour, cocoa, sugar, and espresso powder in a large bowl.

Add the milk, vegetable oil, vanilla extract, and egg to the other ingredients and beat them well using an electric mixer.

Carefully pour boiling water into the electric mixer and mix on low speed until perfectly combined.

Mix on high for about a minute to add some air into the batter.

The batter will appear liquid than what you would expect for normal cakes; this is how it should be.

Evenly add the batter into the cake cases no more than ¾ full.

Place them into the preheated oven and bake for about 15-18 minutes or until the mixture can bounce back when tapped.

When done, remove from the oven and allow them to cool before icing.

For the icing, mix the icing sugar and the butter until pale and smooth.

Add matcha powder mixed with vanilla and stir well again.

Finally, add the cream cheese and mix until smooth.

Spread this mixture over the cakes and serve.

Matcha juice

Preparation time: 5 minutes | Cooking time: 0 minutes| Servings: 3

Ingredients:

½ tsp of matcha powder (or you can use 1 tea bag strongly pre-steeped in a ¼ cup of water, and cooled)

2 handfuls of kale

Handful arugula

2-3 stalks of celery

½ granny smith (green, tart) apple

3 sprigs parsley

½ lemon, but juiced prior

Directions:

Juice the vegetables and fruit.

Squeeze the lemon in afterwards (do not juice it).

Stir in the matcha green tea powder or the chilled green tea afterwards.

Very green juice

Preparation time: 5 minutes | Cooking time: 0 minutes | Servings: 3

Ingredients:

1 kiwi, peeled, halved

½ cup pre-pressed apple juice

½ ripe pear, cored

1 cup baby spinach leaves (pull off stems if you would like)

¼ avocado, pitted and scooped out

Directions:

Simply juice until smooth.

Summer watermelon juice

Preparation time: 5 minutes | Cooking time: 0 minutes | Servings: 3

Ingredients:

½ cucumber, halved

2 cups baby kale (can remove stems if you like)

2 cups of pre-cut watermelon chunks

4 mint leaf

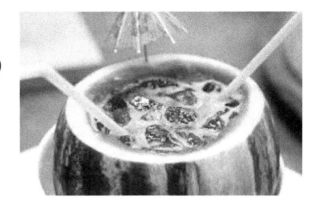

Directions:

Add all to a blender and blend it very well.

Enjoy.

You cannot juice watermelon!

Banana berry smoothie

Preparation time: 5 minutes | Cooking time: 0 minutes | Servings: 3

Ingredients:

1 banana

1 cup blackberries

1 cup blueberries

2 tbsp natural yoghurt

1 cup milk (or soy/almond or rice milk)

Directions:

Add all to a blender and process until smooth.

Matcha green tea smoothie

Preparation time: 5 minutes | Cooking time: 0 minutes | Servings: 3

Ingredients:

2 bananas

2 tsp matcha green tea powder

½ tsp vanilla bean (paste or scraped from a vanilla bean pod)

1½ cups milk

4-5 ice cubes

2 tsp honey

Directions:

Add all ingredients except the matcha to a blender.

Blend until smooth.

Sprinkle in the matcha tea powder, stir well or blend a few seconds more (or add cooled green tea).

Green-berry smoothie

Preparation time: 5 minutes | Cooking time: 0 minutes | Servings: 3

Ingredients:

1 ripe banana

½ cup blackcurrants (take off stems)

10 baby kale leaves (take off stems)

2 tsp honey

1 cup freshly made green tea (dissolve honey first in tea then chill)

6 ice cubes

Directions:

Dissolve the honey in the tea before you chill it.

Cool first, and then blend all ingredients blender until smooth.

Green grapefruit smoothie

Preparation time: 5 minutes | Cooking time: 0 minutes | Servings: 3

Ingredients:

1 grapefruit, peeled and deseeded

6 large kale leaves, destemmed

1 green or red apple, cored and destemmed.

1 carrot

½ cup of water (may use more or less for the texture that you like)

Directions:

Place everything into a blender, and blend until smooth.

Add water if needed.

Green apple smoothie

Preparation time: 5 minutes | Cooking time: 0 minutes| Servings: 3

Ingredients:

1 green apple, cored and destemmed and sliced

6 large kale leaves, destemmed

1 orange, peeled

1 stick of celery

Directions:

Juice the orange separately in a blender and strain, unless you have a citrus juicer/press.

Juice the celery, kale and apple, mix together and stir, or add to a blender and pulse for a few seconds.

Creamy green sunshine smoothie

Preparation time: 5 minutes | Cooking time: 0 minutes | Servings: 3

Ingredients:

1 avocado, pitted and scooped out

1 banana

5 leaves of kale, destemmed

½ cup of pineapple juice

8 oz. of coconut water

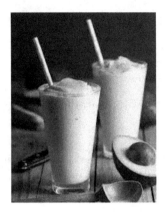

Directions:

Place the liquids then the fruits and veggies into a blender and blend until smooth.

Pizza kale chips

Preparation time: 5 minutes | Cooking time: 40 minutes | Servings: 3

Ingredients:

250g (9oz) kale, chopped into approx. 4cm (2inch)

50g (2oz) ground almonds

50g (2oz) parmesan cheese

3 tbsp tomato purée (tomato paste)

½ tsp mixed herbs

½ tsp oregano

½ tsp onion powder

2 tbsp olive oil

100ml (3½ fl oz) water

Directions:

Place all of the ingredients, except the kale, into food processor and process until finely chopped into a smooth consistency.

Toss the kale leaves in the parmesan mixture, coating it really well.

Spread the kale out onto 2 baking sheets.

Bake in the oven at 170C/325F for 15 minutes, until crispy.

Rosemary & garlic kale chips

Preparation time: 5 minutes | Cooking time: 20 minutes | Servings: 3

Ingredients:

250g (9oz) kale chips, chopped into approx. 4cm (2inch)

2 sprigs of rosemary

2 cloves of garlic

2 tbsp olive oil sea salt

Freshly ground black pepper

Directions:

Gently warm the olive oil, rosemary and garlic over low heat for 10 minutes.

Remove it from the heat and set aside to cool.

Take the rosemary and garlic out of the oil and discard them.

Toss the kale leaves in the oil, making sure they are well coated.

Season with salt and pepper.

Spread the kale leaves onto 2 baking sheets and bake them in the oven at 170C/325F for 15 minutes, until crispy.

Chapter 9: Questions and Answers

What's the reason?

It depends on eating a gathering of nourishments that contain something the creators portray as 'sirtuin activators'. Sirtuins are a class of protein, seven of which (sirt1 to sirt7) have been recognized in people. They seem to have a wide scope of jobs in our body, including potential enemies of maturing and metabolic impacts.

As researchers see increasingly about sirtuins, they're getting keen on the job they may play in assisting with turning on those weight reduction pathways that are normally activated by an absence of nourishment and by taking activity. The hypothesis goes that in the event that you can actuate a portion of the seven sirtuins, you could assist with consuming fat and treat weight with less exertion than it takes to follow some different eating regimens or go through hours on the treadmill.

What does it include?

The sirtfood diet has two phases. On every one of the initial three days, you drink three 'sirt juices' and have one supper (aggregate of 1,000 calories per day). On the accompanying four days, you're permitted two sirt juices and two dinners day by day (aggregate of 1,500 calories day by day). You at that point progress to the simpler stage two, with one juice and three 'adjusted' dinners, in reasonable bit measures, a day.

What would you be able to eat on the eating regimen?

There's a rundown of nourishments containing synthetic intensifies that the creators' state switches on sirtuin and wrench up fat consumption while at the same time bringing down hunger (the last most likely through assisting with accomplishing better glucose control).

Is it compelling for weight reduction?

You ought to get in shape essentially on the grounds that you're eating fewer calories, particularly in stage one. Without a doubt, you may consume fat quicker with this eating routine than with 'any old calorie-confined' plan, and you may feel more full. With respect to the creators' case, this eating regimen is 'clinically demonstrated to lose 7lb in seven days'...

Indeed, it's important that so far the eating regimen has just been tried on 40 sound, exceptionally energetic human guinea pigs in an upmarket rec centre in London's Knightsbridge. The analyzers lost a normal of 7lb in seven days while demonstrating increments in bulk and vitality. In any case, at that point, given the calorie limitations of that first week, weight reduction may essentially be because of the extraordinary decrease in calories.

Further examinations are expected to distinguish the long haul sway on waistlines – and general wellbeing – and to see whether sirt calorie counters keep the pounds off any more adequately than they would on different eating regimens. We don't yet have the foggiest idea what, assuming any, sway the expansion of sirt foods to our eating regimen really has on our weight.

What's more, will anybody have the option to stay with the repetitiveness of juices and limit themselves to nourishments on the rundown (and be glad to dump their typical cuppa for green tea) for all time? With respect to the features that recommend you can appreciate dull chocolate and red wine on this eating regimen – well, truly, it is anything but a green light to expend piles of either!

In the event that you have the funds, the tendency and the stomach for it, I'm very certain it will 'attempt' somewhat for the time being, if simply because it's a successful Directions to confine calories. Furthermore, wine and chocolate aside, the rundown, for the most part, comprises of the very nourishments dietitians and nutritionists suggest for good wellbeing (think products of the soil!).

Regardless of whether it functions admirably enough to make it stand separated from a huge number of weight reduction designs that have trodden this tired way before likewise is not yet clear.

Conclusion

The sirtfood diet promotes fat burning, body detoxification, muscle gain and overall health improvement by tapping into sirtuin, or in other words, activates your very own 'skinny gene'.

Though a relatively new diet, it is proven to be effective and yields fast and safe results. As a bonus, you can still eat chocolate and enjoy drinking wine!

I hope this book was able to help you find a suitable and effective diet regimen that will help you on your weight loss journey.

The next step is to continue what you have started, maintain your ideal weight and to choose to be healthy each day.

The first week might be a challenge for you, but as they say, if you want changes, you need to work for it. I guarantee you that once you start seeing the improvements in your body, you will realize that a little sacrifice is totally worth it.

In addition to the aesthetic changes that you will see, it is actually what is "inside" that really counts. Achieving optimum health is now possible with the numerous health benefits of the sirtfood diet. I promise you that the quality of your life will surely be improved, all it takes is adding those healthy sirtuin-rich foods!

Test out all of the recipes, and follow along with each of the phases with the proper foods and drinks. Follow the two planned stages, phase 1 and phase 2, and you will be guaranteed to enjoy more energy, vitality, a lighter feeling, and on average, about 7 lbs. Lighter on the scale each week.

ENERGY MEDICINE
THERAPY

INTRODUCTION

Living your best life and being your best self is more than just accomplishing all of your goals. It's also important that you can enjoy your life. After all, what's the point if you aren't even happy? There are a few ways that you can help you to **FEEL GOOD NOW**. It'll make your goals all seem worth it. You'll be able to be more positive and have a greater appreciation for life. Enjoying your life will allow you to see more clearly what matters to you and what life is all about. You'll feel free and creative. Of course, you can live your life and hate every moment of it. You can suffer through every day, not liking your life and wishing things were different. Or, you can take steps to make your life enjoyable for you so that you can make the most of it. Practicing gratitude can help you appreciate all that life offers truly, and you may feel more positive as a result. Appreciating yourself, those around you and everything that you encounter can give you some positivity. You may also learn how to focus on the present moment, allowing you to experience the greatest joy. You will live in the moment instead of dwelling on what happened in the past or what might happen in the future. Learning to do what you love can help you to be successful and happy. Often, we think that we can only choose one of these, yet it's important to remember that you can have it all. Finally, you'll learn about how and why to improve yourself constantly. If you remain the same, nothing will happen and you won't experience growth. Enjoying your life also requires you to enjoy change.

Practicing Gratitude

Taking a bit of time every day to practice gratitude can highly benefit you. It's super important to be grateful, thankful, and appreciative of all that life offers. When you practice gratitude, it's hard not to be a positive person. You'll be able to focus on everything that you have instead of everything that you want, which can have a huge impact on you. It'll be easier to find the positive traits of people in your life and to find positivity in everything that happens.

It's quite simple to practice gratitude. It's free, quick, and can even be fun. Just a few minutes a day can make a huge difference, and there are many ways to practice gratitude. You'll be a much more positive person for doing so, you'll feel better about your life, and you'll be much more motivated as well. Additionally, you may choose; however, you would like to practice gratitude. Because there are so many ways to do so, you may switch it up every day. You have many options to choose from, so there must be at least one that works for you.

You may keep a gratitude journal for yourself that you write in every day. You may have a gratitude list that you add to every day. This may even just be a portion of your journal. Simply writing down five things that you are grateful for each day can help you focus on what you love. This is great for the morning, as you can start your day on a positive note. You may also want to consider doing this before you go to bed so that you end the day thinking about what you were grateful for throughout the day. This can leave a better feeling about the day as a whole.

There is so much to appreciate! While outside, notice the beauty of the sky, plants, animals, and nature as a whole. Remember to appreciate your friends. They're the ones that are there for you and that you spend time with. The same is true for family. Before eating, take a small moment to be grateful for the food you have; not everyone gets a choice. Find the good in everything. Pause throughout the day and remember how great life is.

Express your gratitude. Tell others how much you love and appreciate them. Smile more often, especially at strangers; they're people too! Practice random acts of kindness without expecting anything in return. Call up friends and family just to say hello. Volunteer for causes that you're passionate about. Compliment others. Contact those who you haven't talked to in a while. Even spending time with others is a great way to express gratitude. Remember to appreciate the time you have with them. Thank those that serve you in your life. This could be a cashier, a janitor, or a flight attendant. These people are essential to the economy, yet they are rarely thanked for their work. You might make someone's day much better for it. Remember to express gratitude towards yourself. Be grateful for both your strengths and weaknesses, and remember to be grateful that you are alive.

It's also important to appreciate the challenges of life. It can be fairly easy to name all of the positive aspects of life you're grateful for. However, it's important also to remember to express gratitude for challenges and mistakes. They make you who you are.

STRATEGY 1
UNDERSTAND THE CAUSES OF
MOOD DISORDERS AND DEPRESSION

Depression isn't the same as a feeling of sadness. It's a mental illness with a specific set of symptoms that can only be formally diagnosed by a trained medical professional.

To qualify for a diagnosis of depression, you need to experience at least five of the following symptoms for a minimum period of two weeks. One of these symptoms must be either a depressed mood or loss of pleasure.

Symptoms: [xvii]

1. A depressed mood that lasts throughout the day, most days of the week

2. Loss of interest and pleasure regarding everyday activities, including previously enjoyed hobbies

3. Significant (5 %+) and unintentional weight change

4. Difficulty getting to sleep or sleeping too much

5. Feelings of restlessness or feeling slowed down

6. Loss of energy and fatigue

7. Feelings of excessive, inappropriate guilt and rumination over actual or perceived mistakes

8. Trouble thinking clearly, problems making decisions, or finding it hard to concentrate

9. Thoughts of death, suicide, or suicide ideation

Caution!

If you suspect you have depression, or are having thoughts of self-harm or suicide, you need to reach out to a doctor or therapist as soon as possible. Self-help guides can be very helpful, but they aren't a substitute for urgent medical care. You can always come back to this chapter when you have received a diagnosis and have started treatment as per your doctor's recommendations.

What Do Cbt Therapists Believe About Depression?

As you know, CBT is based on the idea that the way we see the world affects our mood and behavior. But how exactly can your thought patterns lead to depression?

Key Concept #1: Self-Schemas

A schema is a set of beliefs and expectations about a person, thing, or scenario. We have schemas about everything.[xviii] For example, most of us have a restaurant schema. Your ideas about going out for a meal in a restaurant include expectations about menus, tables, chairs, servers, food, drinks, and so on.

Although every restaurant has its décor, staff, and food, the basic principles are the same. If you've been to a few restaurants, you have a good idea of what to expect the next time. Schemas are useful because they help us plan ahead and respond to new environments. They help us understand how to behave appropriately around other people.

Just as you have a restaurant schema, you also have a "self-schema." As you may have guessed, a self-schema is a set of beliefs about who you are and how you should act.

Someone with a positive self-schema knows they aren't perfect, but they usually think of themselves as a good human being. On the other hand, people with depression often have negative self-schemas.

If you have a negative self-schema, you may have the following beliefs:

"I'm just not good enough."

"I'll never be successful, and I'll never get anywhere in life."

"Everyone leaves me, and I'll be lonely forever."

Beck thought that difficult childhood events could lead to a negative self-schema. For example, if a young boy is bullied at school for a long time, he may grow into a man who believes everyone hates him.

If you think poorly of yourself, you will be vulnerable to depression. A negative self-schema makes it hard to appreciate your achievements and enjoy relationships because you never quite believe you deserve them. Even when things are going well, you might find it hard to trust other people.

Exercise: Completing Sentences

Sentence completion exercises can help you uncover the negative self-schemas that are holding you back.

In your notebook, complete the following sentences. Don't overthink this. Write the first thing that comes to mind.

"I am the sort of person who…"

"In my experience, the world is…"

"When I think of the future, I think…"

This exercise can be quite illuminating. You might be shocked to discover just how negative your thoughts have become.

Your negative self-schemas might keep you trapped inside a cycle of negative thoughts and behaviors. For instance, if you always think that the future is bleak and that things will never get better, you might not bother to make plans or work toward goals.

Key Concept #2: Faulty Processing & Logical Errors

Negative self-schemas go hand-in-hand with logical errors. Logical errors are self-defeating patterns that keep you trapped in an unhealthy state of mind.

Here are a few of the most common logical errors, also known as "cognitive distortions:" [xix] [xx]

1. Black and white thinking

When we're depressed, we often lose sight that life is neither perfect nor terrible. Instead, we are quick to judge things and people as "bad" or "good," including ourselves. Also known as polarized thinking, black and white thinking keeps you from appreciating the nuances of everyday life.

2. Overgeneralizing

If you tend to overgeneralize, you focus on one poor outcome or event and decide that it's bound to happen again. You assume that a single setback dooms you to a miserable future.

For example, let's say you give a presentation at work. It doesn't go very well. Your boss pulls you to one side and gives you advice on how to improve next time.

A non-depressed person might be a little down or disappointed for a while, but they would probably act on their boss' feedback and even thank them for it. However, someone with depression might assume that all their future presentations are doomed and that their whole professional future is in serious jeopardy because of their poor performance.

3. Fallacy of change

Most of us are guilty of trying to get other people to change. Unfortunately, expecting others to change just to suit your agenda will make everyone unhappy. If you are stuck in this cognitive distortion, you believe that everything in your life will be better if the rest of the world gives in to your demands.

For example, a man might believe that his marriage and life in general will improve if and when his wife joins a gym, works out more, and loses the weight she gained after they got married.

4. Just reward fallacy (or "Heaven's reward fallacy")

As we all know, life isn't fair. However, that doesn't keep us from feeling resentful when things don't go our way. Many people with depression think that if they do everything right and treat others properly, they will somehow be rewarded.

Unfortunately, if you hold this view, you'll be disappointed over and over again. Healthy people know that it's great to try your best, but we don't always have control over the outcome. Other people may treat us well or poorly, and we cannot control their actions.

5. Emotional reasoning

When you're in the grip of intense emotion, logical reasoning can fly out of the window. For example, if something makes you feel upset or scared, you might leap to the conclusion that it must be bad. For example, if a depressed person is nervous about going on a date, they might assume that this means it will go wrong and they probably shouldn't go at all.

6. "Should"

People with depression often use the word "should" a lot, both about themselves and others.

Even if you don't try to tell everyone else what to do, "shoulding" yourself isn't much better. Beating yourself up for not living up to a set of unrealistic or arbitrary standards will keep you locked in a state of self-criticism and depression.

7. Personalization

When you personalize an outcome, you assume that you caused it, even if you have no evidence. For example, suppose that your partner didn't get the promotion they wanted. If your first thought is, "If I'd been nicer lately and less stressed, they would have gotten it, I'm a terrible person!" or something similar, that's personalization. When we're depressed, it feels as though we can't do anything right. Worse, it seems like everything is our fault.

8. Catastrophizing

Also known as "blowing everything out of proportion" or "making mountains out of molehills," catastrophizing involves giving negative events or outcomes more weight than they deserve. When you catastrophize, you conjure up worst-case scenarios, usually in a matter of seconds.

For example, suppose you forget to pick up your partner's suit from the dry cleaner on your way home from work, and only remember once you start cooking dinner. If you are a catastrophizer, you may tell yourself things like, "I'm such an awful partner! We'll get into a fight, they'll leave me, and then I'll be alone forever!"

9. Filtering

When someone is overly optimistic about something, we say that they're wearing rose-colored glasses. If you're depressed, you're wearing gray-tinted glasses instead! If you focus on unpleasant details and ignore the bigger picture, you are filtering.

10. Blaming

People with depression assume that others have the power to "make" them feel a particular way. But this is a fallacy.

Suppose someone insults you. You might feel mildly offended, baffled, outraged, deeply upset, or something else entirely. What determines how you feel? Your approach to the situation. When you blame someone else for your emotional state, you are surrendering your power.

11. Mind reading

Do you assume that you "just know" what someone else is thinking? Do you think you can tell when others are judging you? Mind reading can make you feel depressed, fast. For example, if you tell yourself, "Oh, so-and-so didn't return my email, she must think I'm completely incompetent and is avoiding me," there's a good chance you'll feel bad.

Depressed people are quick to assume that everyone is thinking the worst of them. In reality, most people go through their daily lives thinking only about themselves.

How To Fight It Without Medication

Having depression and all these negative outcomes is not the end to a happy life. The recovery will depend on the course of action you take, though the process is not as easy as you may want it to be. As you start the journey, it is good to note that whatever that seems so complicated can be the best remedy you might ever have! Therefore you don't have to fear trying things out.

The first step towards your recovery is accepting that you are depressed. You also need to understand the cause of your depression and the type of depression you may be having. So, how can you deal with depression?

Take care of yourself

Every healing process starts from you. Of course, the signs and symptoms that you observe may have been caused by some of your actions. The key here is to start diverting your attention away from depression and starting to think about other things that are refreshing. The change of approach will help you eliminate the threat depression is posing in your life.

You can start by setting achievable targets for yourself then working towards attaining bigger goals. The more "small" goals you achieve, the higher the likelihood that you will feel better about yourself. Your goals should include such things like changing your lifestyle, taking a healthy diet, managing the stress levels, following a set schedule to carry out tasks etc. Approach your set goals one at a time spending a little moment appreciating your progress however small it is. Here is a quick summary of some of the goals that you could set to help you in dealing with depression.

How To Overcome

As you read through the list above, did any errors stand out for you? Note that you can be very depressed and only use one or two of these distortions, so don't be surprised if you didn't recognize most items on the list. Over the next few days, challenge yourself to spot your distortions.

1. Healthy Lifestyle Changes To Combat Depression

To ensure a healthy body and mind, you need to adopt a healthy lifestyle. You see, your lifestyle will be the backbone of everything else you do to overcome depression. If you do not fix it, you are unlikely to get any positive outcomes. Coping with depression will be easier if your lifestyle supports a healthy mind and body—because depression attacks the mind and body.

When we talk about lifestyle, what exactly do we mean?

A lifestyle is a way of life established by a society, culture, or an individual. There are elements of a lifestyle that define how you live your life. They include:

- Fitness: Your level of physical fitness and your involvement in physical activities.

- Food: How and when you eat and what you eat.

- Environment: Whom or what is around you, your experience of nature/the world around you, and your impact on it.

- Social life: The state of your social interactions and social fulfillment in areas such as friendship, relationships, community, and family.

- Hobbies and activities: Your pursuit of interests and hobbies. Which ones are they? How involved are you in them?

When we say make positive changes to your lifestyle, the above are the elements we have in mind. If any of them do not support a healthy mind or body, you ought to transform it.

Recommended lifestyle changes to help you overcome depression include:

Food

Eat healthy nutritious food; even though we may not understand this, we are what we eat. What we eat affects us physically, emotionally, and mentally too. Food affects how you feel, your mood, and how you think. Food is fuel, and therefore what you consume determines the kind of fuel powering your bodily system. If you fuel your body with low-quality oil, it will negatively affect its functionality.

For instance, sugar can cause mood fluctuations. You may notice that when you eat a sugary snack, you will experience a sudden spike in energy and positive emotions, what most refer to as a sugar rush. This rush has a very short life span, as a crushing low soon follows it, coupled with a sudden drop in energy and a rush of awful feelings. These energy and mood fluctuations make depression worse.

Experts also suggest that low levels of vitamins, low intake of fatty acids, and mineral deficiencies can lead to an altered mood and mimic mental health issues. In particular, insufficient vitamin D intake may lead to mood swings, lethargic feelings, and depression.

For reasons such as these, you need to consume healthy foods. That means you should consume more of:

- Complex carbohydrates such as whole grains and legumes.
- Fresh fruits and vegetables.
- Fatty acids (omega-3s and omega-6s) to be found in fish, nuts, and olive oil.
- Unsaturated fats such as olive oil.
- Enough water (at least two liters—about sixty-four ounces—a day).
- Amino acid–rich foods.

Limit/cut out the consumption of:

- Sugary drinks with empty calories, such as soda.
- Processed foods with little nutritional value.
- Caffeine.

- High-fat dairy.

- Fried foods.

When it comes to food and diet, the essential thing to keep in mind is to adopt a healthy, balanced diet.

Physical Fitness

The only way to achieve physical fitness is through exercise. Does this mean you should head to the gym and lift massive weights every day of the week? The answer is no. Taking that flight of stairs, parking a little farther from the office, or going for a morning or evening jog or walk counts as exercise.

According to experts, exercise increases the body's production of antidepressants. High-intensity activities such as jogging, running, step dancing, and others trigger the release of feel-good chemicals called endorphins and other hormones that make you feel happier.

Have you ever taken a walk around the block or gone to the gym for a hard workout while stressed? You may have noticed that afterward you seemed to have breathed out all that negativity, your stress reduced, and you were in a better mood.

How and when to exercise

When or how you exercise is entirely up to you. That mentioned, the recommendation is that you should develop a regular exercise routine considering your schedule and everything else on your plate. The exercise regimen must be sustainable and consistent; do not waste your time and energy starting something you cannot stick with—quitting halfway through will have no positive effect on your depression.

When you cannot get started

The physical manifestations of depression, such as reduced energy, disturbed sleep, irritability, and mood swings can result in a lack of motivation to exercise. Understandably, when you are feeling awful, waking up early and going for a jog or going to the gym is unfathomable. It is more comfortable to sleep in and wallow in your sadness. Learn to not listen to your body during such times.

Even when you are not feeling up to it, get up and start small: move a little! For instance, take a five-minute walk around the block, ride a bike, or skip rope for two minutes. The important thing is that you are doing something. Soon, five minutes will grow to ten, and then fifteen, until exercising becomes a big part of your morning routine. The more you exercise, the more you will want to do it because feel-good chemicals are addictive; you will want to feel that good every morning!

Environment

External factors also determine your mental well-being and mood. These factors are within our environment, which is why what is in your surroundings matters. When we talk about the state of your habitat, we are referring to the state of your workplace, your home, your favorite hangout spot, your neighborhood. The sounds, lights, voices, water, and the air around you matters.

Creating a healing environment

The natural environment

- Shield yourself against noise pollution: Trauma is enough noise in your mind. If your mind has to process and filter any more noise, finding peace and tranquility will prove elusive. Noise pollution acts as a parasite on the brain. During this time of healing, you must shield yourself from noise pollution. It is hard to do this if you frequent social places like clubs, marketplaces, malls, and so on.

- Increase exposure to natural lighting: Sunlight/natural light is naturally therapeutic. Experts recommend it as a way to deal with seasonal depression. Additionally, while giving us visual comfort, natural light/the sun is a source of vitamin D, which helps regulate our mood, energy, and mental clarity. We spend an average of eighteen hours a day indoors. Spend some time in the sunlight. If you cannot do so, perhaps because you have work, find a space near a window or move to a well-ventilated area that lets in light.

Work environment

A positive work environment is essential to your mental well-being. If your work environment is not favorable, then overcoming depression may be a little harder.

Work is more than a place where you earn a living. It should provide you an outlet for creative energy and education. Engage in a career you love, or create a positive work environment that gives you a chance to create a healthy work-life balance.

Home environment

Within your home, you are free to create a habitat that fosters your mental, emotional, and physical well-being and health. Try to have more human interactions, which are better for your health than TV and movies. Additionally, interact more with nature.

Social Life

Who is in your life? With which people do you spend most of your time? Where do you spend your time? How you answer these questions sums up your social life, which has a significant impact on your wellness and mental health.

You must maintain healthy relationships. If you keep the company of negative people, developing positive perspectives will prove difficult. If you are in toxic relationships, you will struggle to maintain a healthy mind since you will feel stressed and filled with negativity most of the time.

A healthy relationship is any relationship that has a positive impact on your life positively; such a relationship has mutual respect, love, and understanding. While in such a relationship, you can be yourself, grow at your pace, and you feel respected—and know that you are. Such a relationship is also free from verbal, physical, or emotional abuse and harmful elements like name-calling, hitting, or feeling forced to do unhealthy things.

Create a healthy, balanced social life. Having a social life does not mean you should be friends with everyone or attend every social gathering. Too many social commitments are not ideal for your mental health because they will leave you feeling pulled in too many directions, which will make it challenging to experience peace of mind and sanity. When you continue to put yourself under such pressure, overcoming depression and anxiety will seem too monumental an undertaking.

A healthy social life allows you to have time for yourself to tend to your commitments, quality time to spend with your family, time for your career, and time for your friends.

Limit your social media consumption. We now have a new social life on social media. You want to spend less time on social media, especially when you are dealing with depression. Using social media excessively can lead to negative emotions such as anger, envy, and bitterness.

Most social media posts have an element of showing off; everyone is posting their good moments. On social media, when you are feeling sad about your life, someone else is posting his or her glamorous and super exciting moments, which, even though they may not be 100 percent authentic, will leave you feeling desolate and as if your life is duller than it is.

Hobbies And Activities

Depression may cause you to lose interest in hobbies and activities you may have loved participating in early. If you have activities that made you feel happy and alive, you need to get back to doing them.

Enjoy your hobbies and commit to taking part in the activities you love. At first, you will not want to do it; this does not mean you should sit by the sidelines when you would genuinely enjoy a game of football or experimenting with a new recipe.

STRATEGY 2
UNDERSTAND THE CAUSES THAT GENERATE ANXIETY

ANXIETY AND YOUR BRAIN

Imagine you're enjoying a nice walk through the woods when you encounter a slithery thing on the ground. Light that's reflected off the object will enter your eyes and fall on your retinas, leading to signals that travel through the brain's relay station (the thalamus) and into the primary visual areas located at the back of your brain. The information is then relayed to other parts of the brain, including memory areas that match the object with the concept "snake."

The fact that you're seeing a snake is then passed along to other areas, including the amygdala, tucked deep inside your brain, central to feeling and expressing fear and other emotions. How does your brain know to fear a snake next to your foot on the ground but not the one behind the glass at the zoo? The amygdala also gets input from the hippocampus, which is crucial for understanding context. Thanks to your hippocampus you may even start to feel afraid the next time you walk through the woods, even if you don't run into a snake.

Signals from the amygdala then activate a brain area called the hypothalamus, which will activate the fight-or-flight response of the sympathetic nervous system by releasing stress hormones like epinephrine (adrenaline). The hypothalamus also triggers the pituitary gland to release hormones into your bloodstream that travel to your adrenal glands (which sit on top of your kidneys), causing them to release additional stress hormones like cortisol. Our existence on this planet has depended on this coordinated response, allowing us to recognize and respond to threats, like moving away from the snake.

Just as it's important for our survival to learn to fear certain stimuli, it is also adaptive to learn when danger is minimal so we're not overly fearful. This new learning depends on providing our brains with new information, which anxiety-driven avoidance can prevent. For example, if I always avoid dogs because a big dog knocked me down when I was a little kid, I'll never learn that my early encounter won't be my typical experience with dogs. When we practice mindfulness and cognitive behavioral techniques for dealing with fear and anxiety, we retrain these brain areas to change their response to things that scare us.

Strategies For Working Through Worry, Fear, And Anxiety

There are many tools for managing overwhelming worry, fear, and anxiety, including cognitive, behavioral, and mindfulness techniques.

THINK (COGNITIVE)

When our fear is activated, we're likely to have thoughts that terrify us even more. For example, if we're gripped by fear on a plane, we might become convinced the plane will crash, which further heightens our fear and continues the cycle (refer to the CBT model of anxiety here). By challenging our anxious thoughts, we can interrupt this feedback loop.

A note of caution: when we're overwhelmed with anxiety, it's difficult or even impossible to talk ourselves down with reason alone. These techniques will tend to be most effective before anxiety has taken over and combined with behavioral and mindfulness techniques.

Remember that anxiety is not dangerous. We often come to fear anxiety itself, believing it's dangerous to be too anxious. However, as uncomfortable as it can be, anxiety itself is not harmful. Furthermore, fear about being anxious only leads to more anxiety. Keep in mind even in a severe bout of anxiety that the physical, mental, and emotional symptoms will not hurt you.

Reassess the likelihood of danger. Our fear will convince us that what we're afraid of is going to happen. But keep in mind that anxiety disorders by definition involve unrealistic fears given the actual risk, so the probability that they will come true is quite low. If your fear is telling you something really bad is likely to happen, you can use the Core Belief form to test this belief. How strong is the evidence supporting it? Is there any evidence against it? Has it happened before, and if so, with what frequency? If you discover any errors in your thinking, reevaluate the likelihood that what you fear will happen in light of the evidence.

Reassess the severity of threat. Sometimes the thinking error we make isn't about how likely a negative outcome is but how bad it would be. For example, Joe thought it would be terrible if people knew he was anxious while giving a talk. As he examined this thought, he realized that people might indeed know he was anxious from the quiver in his voice or shaking hands, but realized it probably wouldn't be a big deal. After all, he'd heard speakers who seemed nervous before, and their anxiety hadn't colored his overall perception of the person or the quality of his or her speech.

Why worry? Worrying is a hard habit to break, especially because we often believe we should worry. We might tell ourselves that worrying:

- Helps us think of solutions to a problem

- Prevents us from being blindsided by bad news

- Shows we care

- Can make things turn out well

- Helps motivate us

These beliefs generally are false. For example, we can't avoid potential pain by imagining the worst-case scenario, which would be just as upsetting if it happened—plus we feel needless distress from countless worries that never materialize. When we see the futility of worry, we're more likely to redirect our thoughts.

Test your predictions. This technique sits at the intersection of cognitive and behavioral approaches. When you've identified a fear about how a specific situation will turn out, you can design a way to see if your forecast was right.

Lily dealt with a lot of social anxiety at work. She was convinced that if she spoke up in a meeting, her colleagues would ignore her ideas and probably even criticize them. She wrote down these and other expected outcomes before a meeting, and then she took a risk and volunteered her thoughts. While people seemed a bit surprised when she spoke up, nobody criticized her ideas. Her supervisor asked her to lead a subgroup that would develop her proposal. After the meeting, Lily wrote down the actual outcome versus her prediction.

Our core beliefs can distort our memories, thereby reinforcing our beliefs. It's important to record when our predictions turn out to be false, to help us encode and remember information that's counter to our expectations.

ACT (BEHAVIORAL)

When we change how we respond to situations that make us anxious, we can learn new behaviors that lessen our fear. Let's review some strategies for using our actions to combat our anxiety.

Approach what you fear. Facing our fears head-on is called "exposure therapy" in CBT and is the antidote to the avoidance that maintains anxiety. (This assumes, of course, that what we fear is not very risky; facing a dog that bites won't fix our phobia of animals, for example.) Exposure to the things that scare us decreases our anxiety by:

- Allowing our nervous system to learn that the danger is exaggerated

- Giving us confidence that we can face our fears without being overwhelmed

- Reinforcing our awareness that anxiety is not dangerous

Face your physical manifestations of fear. Anxiety about our anxiety can present an additional challenge. Panic disorder in particular can feature a fear of the panic-related physical sensations. For example, a person might avoid running because the resulting shortness of breath and pounding heart are similar to panic. Avoiding physical sensations only strengthens our fear and makes us more sensitive to the sensations. Exposure therapy can decrease our fear of physical anxiety symptoms. For example, we can do jumping jacks to cause breathlessness, spin in a chair to induce dizziness, or wear warm clothes to make ourselves sweat. Doing these kinds of things repeatedly lessens our fear of the physical sensations.

Let go of safety behaviors. When we have to do something that scares us, we often incorporate behaviors intended to prevent what we're afraid of from happening. For example, if we're afraid of going blank while giving a talk, we might write out and read our whole presentation. Other examples include:

- Keeping our hands in our pockets in social situations in case our hands shake

- Being overly cautious to avoid offending anyone

- Traveling with a companion only because of anxiety

- Triple-checking an e-mail for mistakes before sending it

There are two main problems with safety behaviors. First, they teach us that but for the safety behavior, things would have turned out badly, thus perpetuating the behaviors and our fears. Second, they can impair our performance, as when a capable speaker is overly reliant on notes, which prevents him from engaging with the audience.

In reality, many of our safety behaviors are useless, but we never realize it if we always use them (just like a superstitious practice we're afraid to let go of). We can combine testing our predictions with dropping safety behaviors to test whether they're necessary directly.

Strategy To Overcome

Breathing is characterized as a programmed capacity of the body that is overseen by the respiratory framework and ran by the central nervous system. Breathing can be seen as a reaction of the body when it is faced with pressure, where there is a stamped change in the breathing tempo and rates.

This is a piece of the body's fight or flight system and is a piece of the body's reaction to upsetting circumstances. People have been enabled to control their breathing patterns, and studies have proven that with our capacity to control our breathing patterns we can oversee and battle pressure and other wellbeing related conditions such as depression and anxiety.

Controlled breathing when utilized in the act of yoga, tai chi and other reflection exercises, is likewise used to achieve a condition of unwinding. Controlled breathing strategies can mitigate the accompanying conditions:

- Anxiety issues

- Panic attacks

- Chronic fatigue disorder

- Asthma assaults

- Severe agony

- High pulse

- Insomnia

- Stress

How To Overcome

Mindfulness provides several ways to manage our fears, through both the present focus and the acceptance components of the practice.

Train the breath. Our breath is closely connected to our anxiety: slow and even when we're at ease and fast and sharp when we're afraid. You can feel the contrast right now by first taking a series of fast, deep breaths in and out. Notice how you feel. Then breathe in slowly and out even more slowly. Feel the difference? When we're anxious we often aren't even aware that our breathing is mirroring our anxiety. Once we become more aware of the quality of our breath, we can practice more relaxed breathing:

1. Breathe in gently for a count of two.

2. Exhale slowly to a count of five.

3. Pause after you exhale for a three-count.

4. Repeat from step 1 for 5 to 10 minutes, one to two times per day.

These periods of focused attention on the breath will make it easier to practice relaxed breathing when you need it most. When you feel your anxiety start to increase, practice coming back to the breath.

Focus on the present. Anxiety grabs our attention and pulls it into the future. With practice, we can train the mind to come back to the present. As we disengage from future-oriented fears, we allow anxiety's grip to loosen.

2. Coping With Worrying

Worry is the interest you pay in advance for the loan you may never take out.

Do you always have to deal constantly with worries and anxiety? Here are some useful tips to help ease your anxiety and calm your troubled mind.

How much is too much?

It is very normal to experience worries, anxiety and doubts in daily life. It is our reaction to it which makes the greatest difference in our lives. It's very natural to get worked up about a first date, an upcoming interview, or an unpaid bill. Becoming frequently worried becomes overwhelming when it is uncontrollable and persistent. If every day you become worked up by picture all of the negative things that might happen to you, you are letting anxious thoughts interfere with your life and well-being.

Negative thoughts, incessant worrying, and constantly expecting poor outcomes will have a negative effect on your physical and emotional well-being. It gradually weakens you emotionally, taking your strength and leaving you restless and nervous, with headaches, insomnia, muscle tension and stomach problems.

The effect of this on your personal life, your concentration at school and work cannot be overemphasized. For some people, it's easier to take out their frustration on your loved ones and people closest to them, take alcohol or drugs or try to distract themselves by tuning out from everything.

Chronic anxiety and worry is a sign of Generalized Anxiety Disorder (GAD), a disorder that causes restlessness, nervousness and tension, together with a feeling of unease which can take over your life.

If you feel burdened by tension and worries, you can take a few steps to take your mind off anxious thoughts. Over time, worrying constantly becomes a problem. It becomes a mental habit when prolonged and is very difficult to break. Train your brain to be calm and think only positive thoughts, and change your outlook on life to a more relaxed and confident perspective.

Why Is It So Hard To Quit Worrying?

Worrying constantly does nothing but affect your life negatively. It keeps you up at bedtime and makes you edgy and tense in the daytime. You may detest the feeling of being nervous and confused, but it's very difficult to stop worrying. Beliefs about worrying, either positive or negative, fuel this nervousness further and may cause additional anxious thoughts in chronic worriers.

Negative Beliefs About Worrying

Most people believe that getting worried constantly is very harmful to your health and can drive you nuts. You may be worried about losing control over your thoughts and worries, fearing that they'll consume you and never stop. Negative beliefs about worrying may further fuel your anxiety, but positive beliefs about worrying can do as much harm.

Positive Beliefs About Worrying

You may believe, either consciously or unconsciously, that you can prevent bad things from happening to you, prepare for the worst and foster solutions. Probably, you keep convincing yourself that by worrying about a particular thing for a long time, you'll be able to figure it out eventually.

If you're convinced that getting worried is the most responsible thing to do in such a situation and the only way to avoid overlooking anything, it's even more difficult to break the habit. When you come to the realization that worrying is not the solution but the problem itself, you will be capable of gaining control of your mind.

How To Quit Worrying

Tip 1: Choose a Short Period Each Day to Worry

It can be quite difficult to be productive when your thoughts are consumed by worry and anxiety, distracting your attention from school, work, or your family. In this case, the strategy of putting off worrying can actually do a lot of good. Instead of getting rid of these thoughts, grant yourself permission to have these thoughts later on in your day.

Dedicate a period for worry each day. Set up a time and place to think of things that bother you. It should be at the same time every day (for example, 6 p.m. to 6:15 p.m. in the bedroom). Choosing a timeframe that won't affect your bedtime and or create additional anxiety in your life. During this period, you can worry about whatever you want. The rest of the day should be classified as worry-free.

Put down your worries in writing. When you find yourself thinking anxious or worrying thoughts, simply note them briefly and continue with your daily activities. Always remind yourself that there's time for you to think about it later; there is no need to get worked up about them now.

Tip 2: Challenge Anxious Thoughts

The way that you look at the world may be altered a bit if you are a chronic worrier and thinker. It changes everything, and you may tend to feel threatened. For instance, you picture only a worst-case scenario, and you assume the worst or handle your anxious thoughts as if they were facts.

As a result, you may not feel secure enough to tackle daily challenges head- on; you may assume that you'll lose it at the slightest sign of trouble. Such thoughts, also known as cognitive distortions, include: "All-or-nothing" thinking, having a black-and-white perspective, concluding that "If it isn't perfect, then I'm a complete failure", or "I wasn't hired for this job; I'll never get any job again". You may make a generalization from just one negative experience and expect it to be true forever. Life doesn't work that way.

You may notice only the things that went wrong in your day, instead of things that went well, resulting in thoughts such as: "I didn't get the last test question; I'm stupid, and I can't do anything right.". You may attribute positive events to sheer luck, rather than your own ability to create positive outcomes.

Tip 3: Differentiate the Solvable Worries from the Unsolvable Worries

Studies have shown that you experience less anxiety when you worry. While you think about the problem in your head, you're distracted from your emotions for a while and feel like you're actually solving a problem; in reality, getting worried and problem-solving are two different things altogether.

By problem-solving, you are examining a situation, thinking of solid ways to deal with it, and putting these plans into action. On the other hand, worrying seldom leads to any solutions. The more time that you spend thinking of worst-case scenarios, the less prepared that you are to handle them if they actually happen. That's the simple truth.

Is your worry solvable?

There are different types of worries; some have solutions, while others don't. Solvable worries are those that you can act to resolve instantly. For instance, when you're preoccupied with your debts, you can call a friend or relative to settle your debts, with the option to repay them later.

This type of worry can also be described as productive worry. On the other hand, those worries that do not have a corresponding action can be characterized as unsolvable problems; for instance, thoughts like: What if I get leukemia someday? What if my family gets involved in an accident?

In a situation where you can take action about the thing getting you worried, begin to look for solutions. Compile a list of all the ways you feel that you can solve your worry. Don't get caught in searching for the one perfect answer to the problem.

Concentrate on those things within your reach that can be changed instead of brooding over situations that are out of reach. After deciding upon the solution that will solve your problem, develop an action plan. Immediately you set out to address your fear; you will be less worried.

On the other hand, when the worry is not something you can solve, make peace with yourself by being at ease with the uncertainty. For people who worry excessively, many of their fears tend to be along these lines. People tend to worry when they are trying to anticipate the future, and this is done to feel more in control and prevent potential problems.

However, the bitter truth is that worrying doesn't solve anything; life is occasionally unpredictable. So why not enjoy your life now instead of being engrossed in unpleasant things that have not taken place?

Most people long for inner peace: the feeling that everything is, and will be, all right. But sometimes, we worry, develop fears, and ponder the same things over and over without finding a way out.

The tragic thing is that, of course, we know rationally that the upcoming test is not a life-and-death situation. Our child is probably not lying in the ditch just because he/she does not call at the agreed-upon time. Our dull headache is probably harmless and not the symptom of a brain tumor.

But when our anxiety rises, we think in circles or worry about failing, and we lose that realistic perspective. We are like under a "black cloud". Then we can only imagine all that has happened or is going to happen. We only see what is going wrong in our lives, family, company, and in the world. These thoughts are, in fact, only thoughts — but we lose our perspective.

Do you imagine disastrous, unpredictable things might occur? What is the possibility that these things will actually happen? Even when the probability that bad things will happen is low, do you still worry over the little chance that something terrible will occur?

Tune into your emotions and thoughts and observe them. You can overcome your worries by observing your feelings and thoughts while staying rooted in the present moment. Find out from your loved ones how they combat their uncertainty about things. Can you follow their strategies to overcome your worries?

Tip 4: Interrupt the Worry Cycle

Answer the following questions:

- What am I worried about?

- What possible solutions exist?

- Which solution should I choose?

- How and when do I implement the solution?

Just writing down your worries can provide you with some relief. If you then also write down different solutions, you will see your fears in a different light. You will adopt the observer perspective and will be able to think more logically about what you can do.

Meditate. Meditation helps to alleviate daily worries by shifting our attention. We focus only on the here and now and can leave the concerns of the past or future behind. Similarly, meditation can also help us observe ourselves and understand our negative thought patterns. We only need to find a comfortable, quiet place and focus carefully on our breathing. Various studies have shown that meditating not only helps to ease worries but can also reduce stress and anxiety.

Tip 5: Talk about your worries.

One way to worry less is to talk to our closest friends about what is bothering us. When we are worried, friends can help us to alleviate our fears and see things from a different perspective. They can help us to look at the problem from the outside. Then, we can often find a solution or come to realize that it's not as bad a problem as we feared. When they listen without judgment or criticism and pay attention to what we say, their empathy can help us to feel calmer and more relaxed.

Having someone listen to us with empathy is essential to make us feel better. Even professional help is very beneficial, in some cases, if you cannot find a way out yourself.

STRATEGY 3
UNDERSTAND THE CAUSES THAT GENERATE STRESS

3. Illnesses Caused By Stress

Stress causes many kinds of illnesses that involve both the mind and the body.

You may be battling stress and have some of the health issues and diseases listed here:

Insomnia

Lack of sleep and insomnia exacerbates stress. Worry, uncertainty about the future, issues with your job, your relationships, your children, finances keeps a person awake at night. Some people are concerned with caring for a family member who is ill or a death in the family. Just navigating through each day can raise the level of stress. If stress remains uncontrolled, it interferes or delays the ability to fall asleep.

In order to battle against your lack of sleep that is stress-related, there are positive steps that can be taken. Reduce caffeine intake over the course of the day, stop watching TV or surfing on your computer at least an hour before bedtime, shut off all electronics when you're in your bedroom, and do not exercise prior to bedtime. A bedroom that is dimly lit, cool, and comfortable is the type of environment you want to have before you go to sleep.

Shut your mind off from the problems that elevate your stress while getting ready for bed. Instead, think peaceful thoughts, have soothing sounds or music programmed to play for an hour while you drift off to sleep. Prepare your mind for rest.

Violent or disturbing television programs can elevate stress and anxiety, especially in these days of mass shootings and the traumatic aftermath that people experience from these events.

Depression

Stress that remains unresolved can bring up emotions of anger or hopelessness in a person. Both of these emotions can lead to depression and have feelings prolonged.

Feeling chronically unhappy or sad, having trouble thinking with clarity, dealing with loneliness or feeling unloved and uncared for, or feeling shame or guilt, you are probably depressed, which often is related to excessive stress.

Illnesses you may have that are chronic may seem unrelated to depression. However, continuous daily coping with a chronic condition can be stressful and depressing.

A feeling of hopelessness sets in when a chronic condition is a day-to-day battle. The stress of maintaining the condition with medications, routines that can't be ignored, and the never-ending doctor appointments can be a stressful and depressing way to live.

Disordered Eating And Eating Disorders

When you're feeling stressed and overwhelmed with an issue that you just want to have gone away, do you find yourself looking for something to eat, most often that is tasty and sweet when these feelings well up?

Don't feel like you're alone. That's what many people do.

When people are stressed, they usually reach for a carbohydrate-laden food or a sweet treat to get a fast sugar rush. While your blood sugar may elevate for a short period giving you a false sense of energy, it will drop afterward, frequently making you feel sluggish and, sometimes, drowsy and slow.

There is another eating disorder that stress impacts and that is bulimia. Stress is thought to be an initiator for people who have bulimia and end up binge eating.

Chronic stress and stressful events are major causes of eating disorders. Some research has indicated that the overall pressure and stress for bulimics is more than two times greater than it is for normal women.

The stress may be expressed through anger, anxiety or depression, or physical decline and illness.

Try changing your eating habits when you get stressed out. Eat some crisp veggies like carrots or even raw green or red peppers that have a natural sweetness. Cut up an apple and eat a few slices. You can also pop some light butter popcorn. You'll feel fuller with fiber and stay healthy, as well. Don't allow your stress to have you make a bee-line to the cookie jar, your favorite Danish pastry or candy counter.

Panic Attacks And Anxiety

As with depression, disorders linked to anxiety and panic attacks often have a stress-related correlation.

Struggling with issues that cause you to feel ill-at-ease and have you experience extreme stress and that can manifest in fear and nervousness for reasons that are not clear.

Panic attacks and anxiety attacks are usually thought to be interchangeable. However, they are very different. Although they have some similar symptoms, there are differences that are distinct in how they manifest, how they are triggered, the length of time they last and how each is treated.

It is important to understand how different each attack is so your symptoms can be reported to your physician accurately. Their treatment is different.

The onset of an anxiety attack is different, whereas it is a gradual escalation of emotions. It is usually caused by a particular situation that can be targeted as the cause of the attack.

Symptoms of an anxiety attack before it occurs can be the feelings of worry, uneasiness, fearfulness or distress. These feelings usually begin before the actual attack and continue after the attack ends.

An anxiety attack can last longer than 10 minutes. If a certain situation is occurring that has caused the attack, the anxiety will continue until the situation changes or ends.

Panic attacks, on the other hand, come on instantaneously and spontaneously. This attack is instant. There is no gradual escalation, it just comes at any time, no matter what the situation. There is usually no identifiable reason why the attack occurred.

While you're experiencing the attack, you will experience crippling fear, as well as the fear of losing control. You also have a feeling of disassociation from your surroundings, known as derealization. You may also experience a detachment from yourself, known as depersonalization.

Panic attacks last, on average, approximately 10 minutes. After the attack ends, the symptoms dispel after the attack ends (Boring-Bray, 2018).

Physical symptoms for both attacks:

- Nausea

- Lightheadedness and/or dizziness

- Pains in the chest

- Difficulty in breathing

- Sweating

- Throat tightening or choking sensation

- Physical shaking or trembling

- Tingling or numbness

- Headache

If the panic attacks or uncontrolled anxiety attacks persist or accelerate in their occurrence, meeting with a psychologist or a counselor may be a step in the positive direction of dealing with the source of the issue.

Viruses And Colds

Illness of any kind can cause stress, even if the illness may be a common cold or virus. The immune system that is not functioning up -to-par and is being afflicted by stress will often get sick more frequently and quicker.

Alleviating stress can be helpful in regaining your health and healing from illness much faster.

Circulatory problems

Your body's veins and arteries can be made to tighten up due to stress and the response to the fight-or-flight feelings. Blood flow through the body can be compressed and create further problems such as poor circulation, blood clots or even a stroke.

Get a medical checkup and diagnosis about this type of medical issue.

Local Or Systemic Infections

Emotional or mental stress can delay or interrupt the physical healing of systemic infections, like food poisoning or local infections such as an infected toe/toenail or a splinter that goes unattended.

The body's positive energy is drained due to stress as it attempts to deal with worrying about stress-related problems. There isn't much left by way of energy to sustain the immune functions of the body to heal infectious injuries and illnesses.

Diabetes

Blood sugar that is out of control that is caused by stress is common in those who have diabetes. People diagnosed with diabetes need to eat and maintain a lifestyle that has to regulate their blood sugar levels in prescribed limits. Sugar levels increase or decrease based on the amount of stress a person with this disease is under.

People with diabetes who are overwhelmed and stressed need to monitor their blood sugar levels. If they're on mediation for type 2 diabetes, they need to take their medication, while type 1 diabetics need to monitor their insulin intake. Eating properly is also key to maintaining blood sugar levels.

Heart Problems

Your heart can palpitate, increase the pulse rate and have your blood pressure increase when you are stressed. Stress can put tremendous pressure on the heart and can damage it. Your blood cholesterol can increase by elevated stress levels. Monitor your blood pressure if you are under consistent stress to avert possible strain on the heart.

Exercise and proper eating habits can also help in reducing the stress levels that can affect your heart.

Cancer

Stress that is prolonged can cause chronic inflammation that contributes to cancer risk and exacerbates an already cancerous condition.

Although stress doesn't necessarily cause cancer in itself, all the other health problems that are linked with stress can cause the manifestation of cancer.

Overeating, smoking, and drinking alcohol in excess all can elevate the risk of developing cancer. These habits can develop and be stress-related.

Studies have shown that there are links between certain types of cancers and stress. The body's immune system is suppressed by stress; a person who is battling ongoing stress may not be able to fight against a major illness like cancer.

Other studies indicate that the recurrence of cancer can be affected by stress and fear of cancer returning. The production of the hormone cortisol occurs when the body is stressed for a period of time. This can inhibit the immune system of the body and make it more prone to the recurrence of cancer. (University of Rochester Medical Center, 2007)

New homeopathic treatments such as musical and relaxation therapy are now being included along with the medical treatments for cancer patients. These treatments can help to lessen and ward off the stress that the disease creates and reduce the side effects of the medical treatments prescribed that can be physically overwhelming.

Post-Traumatic Stress Disorder (PTSD)

This disorder develops in those who have had a trauma either directly or indirectly affect them. They suffer from functional impairment or distress for a period of time, usually a month at minimum and some who have been exposed to extreme trauma for the remainder of their lives.

The symptoms of PTSD include experiencing the traumatic again, evading reminders of the trauma, elevated anxiety and negative feelings or thoughts. Mass shootings, natural disasters, terrorist attacks and cities that are under siege have added to the burden of PTSD. Now global in scope and affects 4-6% of the world's populations, the major portion of traumas are associated with sexual or physical violence and accidents.

There is no known cure for PTSD and the treatments that are currently used to help those who suffer from trauma are not effective for all patients.

There is evidence that Vagus nerve stimulation (VNS) may be an aid that is beneficial when added to other exposure-based therapies. The Vagus nerve serves as a connection to the brain from the peripheral autonomic nervous system.

It communicates with the brain and sends a signal at times when heightened sympathetic activity is activated. The Vagus nerve counteracts the sympathetic nerve response. (McIntyre, 2018)

Declutter Your Mind For Reducing Stress

Clearing of the mental clutter is the only sustainable way to have a stress-free and meaningful life. When your mind can think clearly and make decisions based on priorities rather than instincts, your life becomes easier.

These days, the stress in life has increased so much that people have started thinking that peace is the goal of life, it isn't. Peace is the way of life and leading a meaningful and constructive life should be the goal. Even the animals and birds that do not have the same cognitive abilities lead a peaceful life. There is no reason for this life not to be peaceful or be chaotic until some external force is applied.

Think of young kids for that matter. They lead a peaceful and happy life. You need to apply force to make them unhappy. They are beaming with life. But, as we grow, we become gloomy, stressful, and sad. The person doesn't change. It is the clutter that gets accumulated in mind and brings the change in attitude.

If you closely look at the life of a child:

- A child has easy goals

- A child has clear priorities that bring happiness

- A child has easy decisions to make

- A child has few things to compete for

As you grow all these things change for you. You set unrealistic goals for yourself. Your priorities are complex and most of the times have no bearing in present. The number of choices in your life increase causing a lot of indecisiveness. This leads to anxiety, unhappiness, and stress. You increase the competition for yourself. Your mind starts raising the bar on its own. The more cluttered your mind is, the tougher your life will get.

The reason for most of our stress is unconscious decision taking. It is a result of a cluttered mind where decisions are mostly based on trends or instincts. Becoming mindful of our decision-making process and decluttering the mind can help in solving most of these problems.

We are more focused on living a full life rather than living a fulfilling life. We are running in a mindless race to gather material possessions not knowing their use or worth once we have gained them. We waste our lives running after success only to realize in the end that it wasn't worth the pain anyway.

We work for numerous hours in offices. We sacrifice our precious time in looking at the files and miss the smiles blooming on the lips of our toddlers. This is a great loss that can have no compensation in terms of monetary gains.

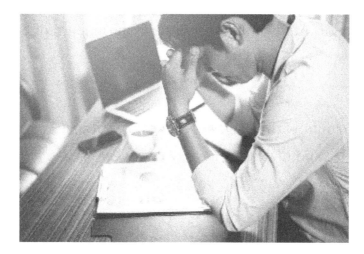

We bear great stress in form of responsibilities. We slog for endless hours in jobs, only to realize that we don't even have the necessary passion for the job. All these things increase stress in life. These are mindless activities are carried out without giving much thought.

This endless talk about not focusing on work and career entirely for money or searching for passion may look a little offbeat. To a materialistic mind, it is a bit off the track. However, it doesn't make the fact any less sad that we are ready to exchange happiness and joy in life in exchange for stress and worthless material possessions.

You work day and night to get rich. You have more than 1 home, more than 1 car and money that is only of any value to you in bank statements. But, you are skeptical to work for something that can give you real gratification.

If you think that searching for happiness in place of material wealth is a difficult and absurd phenomenon, then you are wrong. Not only a person but a whole nation has shown to the world that it is possible and holds merit.

Some major areas have a deep impact on your happiness. If things are neglected in these areas, they automatically lead to stress. Prioritize and see the things you want to have in these areas:

Health

While planning for life, most people never even give a fleeting glance at the health. While we are young, we take it for granted that we'll always be young, healthy, happy and energetic. This notion precipitates pretty fast and we have nothing else to do other than sulk. Health is one of the most important factors that affect our happiness and stress. If you are consciously planning for a stress-free life then leaving health out of that plan is unjust.

Chart out a definite plan for health and fitness. Decide the amount of time and effort you want to give to remain healthy.

Career

We spend the highest amount of time and energy at our workplace. We study, learn, and gain experience to have a stable and rewarding career. But, what use is a career that only keeps you aggravated and dissatisfied? It may give you the money, but that money is only good for boosting your ego and buying stress relievers.

A career should always be rewarding. Something that fuels your passion so that you can become more productive. Do not choose a career that makes you feel miserable. It will make you a part of the rat race.

Work is an important part of life. Yet, it is only a part of life and not the whole of it. If you start compromising with your life for work, in the end, you'll be left with very few things to remain happy. Your work life must have a balance. The amount of work you take must be based on the amount of work you can do. Succumbing to peer pressure, competition and greed may snatch away your happiness.

Relationship

Relationships are important as they complete us. They bring a sense of inclusion in life. However, expectations in relationships and especially unrealistic expectations can turn them toxic. Have a clear idea about the things you want in a relationship. Have a clear, frank and open dialogue about it while entering into a committed relationship. Be more open, accepting and inclusive.

Family

The family is something we easily push aside while making important decisions. The family has its place in life and it should be clear in your mind while you make your decisions.

Self-Improvement

The best thing about us human beings is that we have an indefinite potential for improvement. We can learn new things, languages, arts, craft and make ourselves better. Continuously work on making yourself better. Either it is developing your personality or learning new things, it will make you feel more satisfied. Nothing gives a greater sense of joy than the accomplishment of learning new things. It will keep stress low in your life.

Life Planning

Security is important in life to alleviate unnecessary stress. Planning for life reduces mental clutter. Things move in a more organized manner. You get more time to devote to yourself rather than worrying about the unknown contingencies. Plan things like budget, work, retirement, etc. well in advance.

Recreation

Enjoyment has a special place in life. It gives you joy and pleasure. The end goal of most of the above pursuits is to bring joy to your life ultimately. You must always have space for leisure in life. Plan recreational activities as you plan your work and budget. The moment you start neglecting recreation, stress starts going up.

Cherish Moments

Most importantly, start appreciating life for its merits. Find time to praise life, nature and all the things that fill you with happiness. If you like something, then take out time to look at it more attentively. If anything attracts you, then pursue it.

Living life consciously is the beginning of starting your journey towards leading a stress-free life. Remain mindful of the life around you.

The Role Of Habits In Reducing Stress And Mind Clutter

Clutter at the physical, emotional, or psychological level causes stress. It is one of the biggest reasons for stress.

The physical clutter is obvious. Any excess material that's of no use to you is clutter. Anything that may have been used a long time ago but hasn't been put to use for more than a year is clutter.

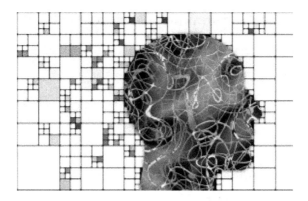

Clearing Physical Clutter is Easy

Clutter takes up space and energy. It uses up your productive energy and distracts you. Your focus can keep deviating if there is clutter around you. Clutter always reminds you that there is one job left to be sorted and you haven't done it. It has a great impact on your functioning and efficiency. You can sort physical clutter by simply removing the unnecessary items from your vision. You can make the system and workplace leaner and things would be better.

Strategy To Overcome

Think of Others Who are in Need:

Take time in your life to stop and give thought to others in the world that is in dire need of help. Many people in the world suffer terribly not knowing where or if they will have a meal each and every day. They have no proper homes, no clean drinking water many die each and every day from ailments that they didn't have to die from. If they only had food and clean drinking water to sustain them like you have. These are people that would gladly trade places with you who have a home, food and clean drinking water but yet you are still unhappy.

Sometimes it takes looking at what others do not have to realize how much you do have and how blessed you are to have the life you have. It may not be your perfect idea of a life but that is up to you to make choices that will improve the quality of your life. At least you have the freedom and options to make choices for yourself many do not have the freedoms you have.

Stop Feeling Sorry for Yourself:

Instead of going on a self-pity trip perhaps you should instead try and focus on more positive things. When you feel yourself going into a depressive state where you think you are so hard done to stop and take a moment to think of all the people in the 3rd world countries that are dying of starvation each and every day while you sit feeling sorry for yourself.

Take this time and use it in a positive way such as making a donation to a charity either financial or by giving your time. You will feel much better than you would just lie around your home buried deep in a self-pity trip. You must get up and dust yourself off and begin taking actions in your life that will lead you to that happier life you seek but just remember to think about those who are less fortunate while doing so.

How To Overcome

However, things are not as easy with mental clutter. Our mind is processing thoughts 30 times faster than the fastest supercomputer in the world. It handles more than 1016 processes in a second. Even when you are not thinking about it, your mind is continuously taking decisions.

For instance, take lunch one afternoon:

You are still in your cubical punching keys on your computer. But, as soon as your mind gets a fragrance of food, it starts thinking about it. The mind doesn't think in a restrained manner. It goes full throttle.

There are thoughts of things you want to eat at lunch, you would want but can't have. Would you be able to get a specific item in the lunch? Would it taste good? Would someone accompany you?

Most of the times, you are not even paying attention to it. Your active participation isn't even required. Your mind is capable of thinking all these in-between things. However, one thing that makes this a problem is that this thinking requires decision making. There are choices to be made.

Whenever there are choices to be made, your mind gets stuck. This activity requires your active participation. The mind wouldn't simply stop at giving you the choices but would question your decisions. This creates a dilemma and any kind of dilemma or hesitation will lead to mental clutter.

You are making thousands of such insignificant decisions in your day. Your mind keeps coming at the points where it requires a decision. It questions those decisions. It debates on the success or failure of those decisions. All this leads to the generation of mental clutter. Any kind of clutter will bombard your mind with excessive stimuli. Your mind would go on an overdrive. There will be unnecessary distraction and hesitation. There will be the physical, mental, and emotional stress of making such decisions. Your mind constantly keeps receiving messages that there is still work pending. It never comes to rest leading to fatigue. It creates anxiety and you may also feel the guilt or repentance of taking decisions. It inhibits your creativity, productivity, and problem-solving abilities. Countless activities of similar nature are running in the background.

All this leads to stress. If it continues for long, it converts into chronic stress and takes a toll on health. This is why people sitting at the position of great power start looking haggard and aged much earlier.

4. Secret To Dealing Your Stress And Anxiety For Good

Mental toughness is a state of being that pulls together a variety of skills, focus, and self-restraint to overcome adverse situations, setbacks, emotional upheaval, and stress/anxiety in order to accomplish a given goal. It is a type of sought-after "superpower" of sorts that most highly successful people have in abundance.

Stress, anxiety, worry, and defeatist attitudes prevent us from achieving our goals and reaching our highest potential. We freeze in our tracks and allow setbacks to define pivotal moments and recall past damage to justify future lack of progress. Mental toughness is about overcoming all the obstacles that we either place before ourselves or are placed before us. It involves learning to cope with life's challenges in order to succeed.

This gives you an edge in your professional life, personal life, love life, athletic activities, and basically anything else you can think of that requires more than a pulse. Put simply, mental toughness makes you more prepared for life.

Think about your ancestors who lived in a world without all of our modern comforts that not only make life pleasant but also safe. They didn't have cozy, cushy lives that protected them from any trace of harm. They couldn't avoid pain because it was a part of life. They displayed the epitome of mental toughness. Hunter/gatherers had to set out into the forest despite the dangers in order to live as well. If they allowed themselves to break down or get taken over by fear, they'd be dead.

Mental toughness is in your head, not your genes, and it certainly doesn't depend on your physical stature. Physical 'toughness' doesn't have to accompany you physically—you can never have set foot in a gym and still be mentally tough. All you need is the "just do it" mentality that Nike has so successfully marketed.

Can anyone develop mental toughness? Yes, it is possible if you take the time to find out what are the obstacles that cause you to fall off the track or not hit the mark. You can cultivate the same skill that the top echelon achievers naturally possess or so it appears.

How the Mind Works

The physical and electrical processes that take place inside the brain structure are relatively complex but are uniform in nature to every human. Differences and aberrations in the features of the brain can cause some differences in response, ability to fire neurons and give adequate reactions.

Energy use of the brain

A group of ambitious researchers at the University of Pennsylvania set out to determine some of the little-understood workings of the brain and its use of energy both at rest and during heavy use.

The first order of business was to come up with a baseline for determining how much the use of energy increased when doing any type of activity beyond rest. The measurement of oxygen used in the brain during activity was the simplest to measure. It turns out that the brain uses the maximum amount of energy in maintaining the firing of electrical energy throughout the brain. It never increased due to an increase in physical activity or thinking.

The good news with these results is that when you have the energy available to be in an awake state means that you have plenty of energy to tackle any thought-driven process or activity.

Alertness and peak activity potentially happen at the midway point of a standard wake period, which varies by the individual.

Distraction potential

In the mid-1980s, a group of clinical psychologists at Michigan State University performed an informal study that involved 60 students conducting a variety of simple tests to determine the basis of brain activity. These students were given an essay to read with a brief questionnaire to answer after. One-half were told to ring a small bell during the time they were reading the essay. The other half were asked to ring the bell during the time period of answering the questions. Those that rang the bell during the reading portion were unable to answer as many questions correctly.

The takeaway on this portion of the informal study is that humans seem to become more distracted during a "thinking" or preparation phase of a project. Those ringing the bell during the answering phase increased their speed in answering correctly. It points to an appreciable line to draw in the sand to eliminate the bad effects of distraction.

It is okay to talk to yourself!

Most people feel self-conscious when talking to themselves, especially if they notice that people are staring and wondering why they are doing it. You will feel good the following time someone tries to discredit you for talking to yourself. The human mind responds far more to verbal cues than quietly trying to remember something. It can be a quick way to move an item in your mind from the short-term to long-term memory storage.

Thoughts, Emotions, and Actions

The development of mental toughness will demand that your thoughts, emotions, and actions are reigned in and kept under tight control during the worst of situations and conditions. Exercise your skills to the point that jumping these hurdles can be as simple as breezing over physical hurdles for skilled athletes.

The basic way that the brain is designed and operates gives you leverage to develop a strong mental toughness for any situation. You can make a mental choice to develop the skills that will propel you towards success or remain quietly living in the background and feeling bitter that nothing about your life changes.

How natural brain activity benefits thoughts

Spending quality time thinking about solutions to problems or making plans to resolve issues seems to be draining and requires tons of extra energy. The truth is that you are using no more energy to think through things than what it takes to be in a waking state. Shake off the feelings of fatigue and understand that your mind is designed to do this effectively. Push past the barriers that are established over false thoughts that make you think that you do not have the energy to make changes in your life.

Distractions and emotions

Being in touch with your emotional side is critical to developing mental toughness. Knowing when emotions are trying to formulate and take over is the perfect time to introduce distraction techniques. You can easily learn how to pull yourself out of an emotional funk that keeps you bound up and unable to move forward. Mental weakness is rewarded through being pliable to raw emotion. It doesn't mean that you have to switch your emotions off completely. You can be a compassionate, feeling person that is not ruled by emotions.

The symbiotic relationship between the brain and body

The ability to formulate the right thoughts, distract to remove emotions, and actively give ourselves verbal instruction demonstrates the symbiotic relationship between our mind and body. Using the natural functions of the brain to your advantage to create a strong sense of mental toughness makes it a method that is both easy and takes a small amount of time to see positive results. You will be able to define your areas of weakness and strength right away. Shoring up your weaknesses will provide you with a stronger foundation for further mental toughening skills development.

Nature and Nurture

What are the factors that determine the way our brains are used? Are we more of a product of our environment or at the mercy of the natural tendencies inherent to all individuals? The short answer is that it is always a combination of both. Striking a balance of good qualities from nature and nurturing is the key to successfully reaching a state of ultimate usable mental toughness. You can retain a sensible approach to life that allows you to maneuver obstructions and obstacles easily.

Identifying negative natural tendencies

Every person has individualized ways of thinking about things and coming to conclusions. Often, these are influenced by natural tendencies or processes that are undergone without any preparation or thought. A few of these are:

- Not wanting to draw attention

- A desire for lack of any conflict

- A desire to not feel negative emotions

- Need for an easy solution

- Consistent problem avoidance

Knowing that you lean toward these natural tendencies can help alert you to seeing how this is affecting the way to think about and process situations. It can help motivate you to push away from a tendency not to think about a problem or look for the simplest solution. Mentally tough individuals are more likely to look for a solution that provides a concrete and fair outcome. You should never avoid thinking about a problem because it brings in negative feelings or causes you to deal with difficult emotions.

Identifying learned behaviors

Non-productive behaviors in our thinking and processing of events can also come from our nurturing and environment. A few examples of this are:

- Being raised in a household with indecisive parental figures

- Having people around that are highly-emotionally charged

- Not addressing situations or problems at all

- Leaving the solutions open-ended to try and please everyone

Being a people-pleaser and unwilling to confront emotional decisions can take you further away from a state of mental toughness than anything else. Tough situations sometimes call for tough decisions. You need to develop these skills if you have been raised in an environment that focuses on trying to make all parties happy. In the end, you will consistently feel like you sold out and are never satisfied with the progress made in life. Mental toughness can be achieved without feeling like you have been heartless, cruel, or discounted the feelings of others.

Turn Negative Thinking Into Positive Thinking

Rewiring your negative thoughts into positive thoughts is all about changing your thought processes. The shift can be intentional or coincidental.

The former way allows you to take control of the thinking process to move towards your goal of positive thoughts. Rewiring your attention to a more positive point can prompt you to be happier. For intentionality to be effective, one needs to be specific on turning their negative thoughts into positive ones.

Practically speaking, you can do this by connecting formerly negative experiences with positive expectations. An example is changing your thought process from considering a scenario that would cause you to be anxious to one of being an opportunity to improve. Adjusting responses to situations could turn situations into positive ones. The act can be a form of building a growth mindset. You may also choose to avoid thoughts that have negative consequences like depression. Such feelings can lead to negative neuroplasticity as they encourage the formation of detrimental mental connections. The result may be a worsening of the effects of negative thought patterns through the development of a negative feedback loop system.

Embracing a growth mindset can assist in developing a higher capacity to endure adverse events. Such a mindset can lead to an increase in perseverance. Adopting a relaxed viewpoint can further support the process of turning thoughts from negative to positive.

Learning cognitive skills can aid your process of rewiring your negative thoughts into positive ones. These skills will provide you with a framework for handling varying considerations that accompany or occur as issues arise.

A healthy lifestyle does play a role in rewiring your thoughts from negative to positive. Choose diets that support brain function.

CPSIA information can be obtained
at www.ICGtesting.com
Printed in the USA
LVHW061055090621
689781LV00003B/281

9 781802 857184